# Stories from the Front Line

## The People Behind the NHS Headlines

**Yvonne Bennett**

*Independent Researcher*

and

**Christina Stead**

*Independent Researcher*

Series in Sociology

VERNON PRESS

www.vernonpress.com

*In the Americas:*
Vernon Press
1000 N West Street, Suite 1200,
Wilmington, Delaware 19801
United States

*In the rest of the world:*
Vernon Press
C/Sancti Espiritu 17,
Malaga, 29006
Spain

Series in Sociology

Library of Congress Control Number: 2024944718

ISBN: 979-8-8819-0104-2

Also available: 979-8-8819-0062-5 [Hardback]; 979-8-8819-0101-1 [PDF, E-Book]

Cover design by Vernon Press. Background image by Freepik.

"The NHS will last as long as there are folk left with the faith to fight for it."

*Aneurim Bevan*

# Table of Contents

# List of Figures and Images

**Figures**

**Images**

# Acknowledgements

Dedicated to our parents.

We would like to thank those who took the time to meet with us and tell their stories.

To Roseanne MacKee, Tracy Jackson, and her daughter Jamie-Lee, we are grateful that you felt able to share such traumatic personal experiences with us. That you chose us to recount the events leading up to and from the deaths of much-loved parents is a great honour. We hope we have made their memories proud.

To the staff who showed real courage and trust in speaking to us, we could not have written this book in such depth without you.

To Alan Bennett, the articles you sent us from local newspapers were of great interest and use. Thank you for reaching out to us, your help was invaluable.

Finally, a huge thanks to Anna Davis and Inge Fleming, who gave up their time to proofread for us.

# Introduction

Yvonne Bennett

This book was inspired by a distressing incident I had with my elderly mother, which I decided to document on the social media platform TikTok. The first video went viral overnight, and within hours I was receiving messages from others who had similar stories to tell. The reasons behind people using social media to chronicle events, be they traumatic or celebratory, will be examined in further detail in a subsequent chapter. My response to the received messages was to write about these experiences as I wanted to give the people who had reached out to me a voice and to see if analysis could explain why so many of our elderly were being let down by the National Health Service (NHS) during medical emergencies.[1]

Despite the title of this book, we were mindful not to fall victim to "'[t]he let down by the NHS syndrome", as labelled by McLardy-Smith (2022, p. 34). We want to investigate the ways in which the public might be failing the NHS, a national institution, in addition to the challenges the NHS faces in providing free care at the point of contact in the twenty-first century. This societal shortcoming may be through unrealistic expectations or by a simple misuse of services.

The UK media reports stories, such as my mum's, with "nauseating frequency and relish" (McLardy-Smith, 2022, p. 34), yet our stories are more than just a headline or tomorrow's fish and chip wrapper.[2] A Google search revealed an abundance of media headlines, a fraction of which are noted below. I must point out that these stories are from across the UK, the final one being my mum's story:

- 21 Jan 2020 — Great-grandmother, 83, died from sepsis after waiting five hours for an ambulance and then 70 minutes to be seen in 'bedlam' A&E, inquest hears.

- 20 Oct 2021 —A great-grandma, who's 87 years old, was forced to wait almost nine hours for an ambulance, lying on her drive in the pouring rain, after falling over.

---

[1] To avoid copyright infringements, we have paraphrased all TikTok comments used in the book.

[2] This is a term which relates back to a time when take away fish and chips were sold wrapped in old newspapers.

- 19 Aug 2022 — Family of man, 87, who waited 15 hours for ambulance say the system is 'broken'.

- 22 May 2023 — A UK grandmother died alone and in agony, as she waited five hours for an ambulance to rush her to a hospital that was only a five-minute drive away.

- 26 Oct 2022 — A *great-grandmother* who fell and suffered a stroke *waited* more than nine *hours for an ambulance* to arrive, her family claims.

- 6 Dec 2022 — Cancer patient, 85, is left lying on patio in the rain for SEVEN HOURS as he waited for an ambulance after a fall - despite living just yards from Welsh hospital.

- 15 Aug 2022 — Glasgow great-gran endured five hours 'screaming in agony' on care home floor waiting for an ambulance.

If, as McLardy-Smith's book title infers "Eden [NHS] is Burning" then perhaps the data collected from the experiences of this book's participants may help douse the flames. Although we will discuss different solutions proposed by various health professional organisations, politicians, as well as those working in the NHS, we do not purport to offer a definitive answer to the difficulties facing this national institution, we cannot extinguish those flames completely. Any NHS reform is a political *hot potato* and, as such, the mere mention of change is met with public hostility and concern.

Not all experiences with the NHS are negative, both Dr Stead and I, have had positive experiences. The following is a conversation from Jordan's interview transcript. I am discussing two local hospitals close to me in Kent and then mention a third that has a poor reputation, yet Dr Stead replies with a different experience:

> **Yvonne**: I think, where I am, I am lucky. We've got two hospitals we can go to... the care is good. We have choices. I've always had good experiences although there are flaws. What is that one up at...? **** you wouldn't go there.
> **Christina**: Except they've treated my husband very well, so....
> **Jordan**: You don't get to hear the stories like that. It's all bad....

If you search for "positive NHS stories," it appears that many NHS Trusts are publishing *feel-good* stories and news pieces on their websites to counter the abundance of negative news. It is not all bad, yet the media focuses on bad news as it is what has historically sold papers. The old newspaper saying *if it bleeds it leads* continues to this day. Is this because people are drawn to news that may affect their lives? Is there a fundamental need to have information to hand that may negatively impact us? As Cohen reminds us, when discussing

NHS111 "[t]he service has not been without criticism, but as Laura Tweedy, an experienced claims handler remarked," [y]ou are always hearing the bad stories and there is little focus on the good stories – and believe me they do exist'!" (2020, p. 51); they are just harder to find.[3]

Using social media to share news may have a different psychological impact on individuals, as it has been suggested that people are drawn to more positive stories and that they use social media as their positive news source (Huffington, 2015). Yet, in my experience, my bad news post went viral while my uplifting content material, such as my sons' weddings or a positive update on my mother's health, garnered only a fraction of the views, likes, and comments. We know the TikTok platform is customised and algorithm-centric, and I can't be the only one who has fallen down a rabbit hole of negative news. Could it be that despite people saying they want to hear good news, they are still drawn to the bad? My sons' weddings have no impact on people's lives, yet my mum's story drew a lot of comments from people with similar stories to tell, people who have been impacted or could be impacted similarly in the future.

This book looks at NHS Scotland with a particular focus on the new Queen Elizabeth University Hospital (QEUH) in Glasgow as this was where the experiences of both me and the participants occurred. Although the attention is on NHS Scotland, we must make it clear that we have utilised research papers that examine NHS services in both England and Wales as well as health care provision in other countries that have a similar free at-the-point-of-contact approach to health care. Although health is a devolved matter in Scotland, just like NHS England and NHS Wales, it is paid for by taxation and a block grant from the UK Central Government.

The primary theme of this book is geriatric care and experience and the risk the elderly face with iatrogenic disease. Iatrogenic disease refers to any disease or injury sustained by a patient which has inadvertently been caused by health professionals within their practice. We, therefore, begin by setting out how we have fixed the age parameters when defining the label elderly as well as examining our understanding and use of the term iatrogenic disease. As noted by Permpongkosol "[t]he definition of the term *elderly* varies widely in medical literature, the most common lower limits being 60,65,70,75 and 80 years of age" (2011, p. 77). We have chosen to use a lower parameter and apply 65 years of age in our elderly definition. We chose to do so after examining national statistics relating to life and healthy life expectancy in Scotland.

---

[3] NHS111 is a 24-hour medical helpline for those who require assistance, but it is not a 999 emergency. The patient is assessed and then directed to the best route of care, be that a GP, pharmacist, minor injuries unit or A&E.

Scotland has the lowest life expectancy in the UK (National Records of Scotland, 2023, p. 2). Life expectancy was shown to be "76.6 years for males and 80.8 years for females in 2019-2021" (2023, p. 3). However, it must be noted that life expectancy in Glasgow City, a deprived area of Glasgow, was three years younger for males and two years younger for females than the Scottish average and six years younger for males and five years younger for females compared to UK data (National Records of Scotland, 2023).[4] We did not solely consider life expectancy when deciding on our age parameters but also looked at healthy life expectancy.[5]

In the 2022 report by National Records of Scotland it was noted that the healthy life expectancy for males was 60.9 years and 61.8 years for females, however, in the most deprived areas of Scotland the healthy life expectancy age "was more than 24 years lower" (2022, p. 5) for both sexes. UK data shows healthy life expectancy ages of 62.8 years for males and 63.6 years for females (Office for National Statistics, 2022).

The health of the UK population is a cause for concern with it now "lagging behind that of many compatible countries." (McKee et al. 2021, p. 1980). The Scottish Government has also highlighted problems the country has "life expectancy and healthy life expectancy trends in Scotland have not improved since around 2012.... This has meant that life expectancy has actually been decreasing for the Scottish population living in the most deprived 40% of areas." (Scottish Government, 2021). In a subsequent chapter, we will discuss what David McCrone has termed "the Scottish effect and the Glasgow effect" (2017, p. 123) this is the phenomena of an increase in levels of disease and death within Scotland and Glasgow.

---

[4] When looking at the UK statistical data it must be noted that the figures include Scotland, and its lower life expectancy and lower life healthy expectancy brings the overall age down. Life expectancy, as noted by McKee. (2021) "has consistently been higher in England than the other three nations with Scotland lagging far behind" (p. 1981).

[5] "Healthy life expectancy (HLE) is an estimate of the number of years lived in 'very good' or 'good' general health, based on how individuals perceive their state of health at the time of completing the annual population survey (APS)." (National Records for Scotland, 2022, p. 6).

**Figure I.1** Life Expectancy in Years.

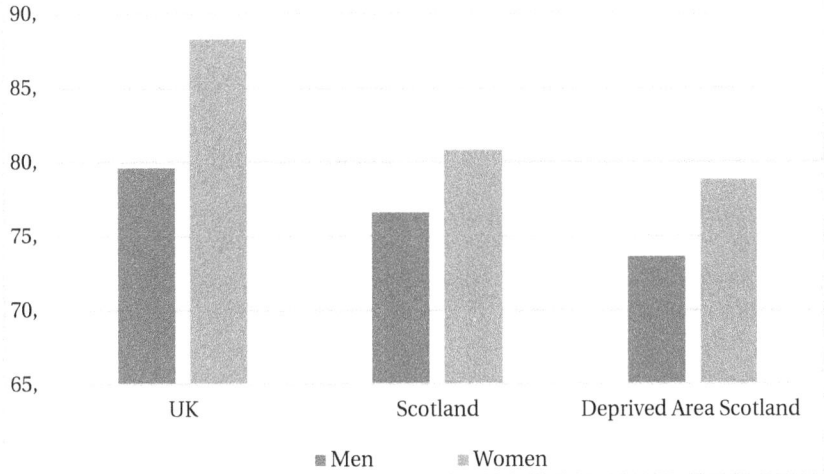

Data from: National Records of Scotland (2022) *Healthy Life Expectancy 2018 - 2020.* Available at: https://www.nrscotland.gov.uk/files/statistics/healthy-life-expectancy/18-20/healthy-life-expectancy-18-20-report.pdf. Accessed: 20th August 2023.

**Figure I.2** Healthy Life Expectancy in Years.

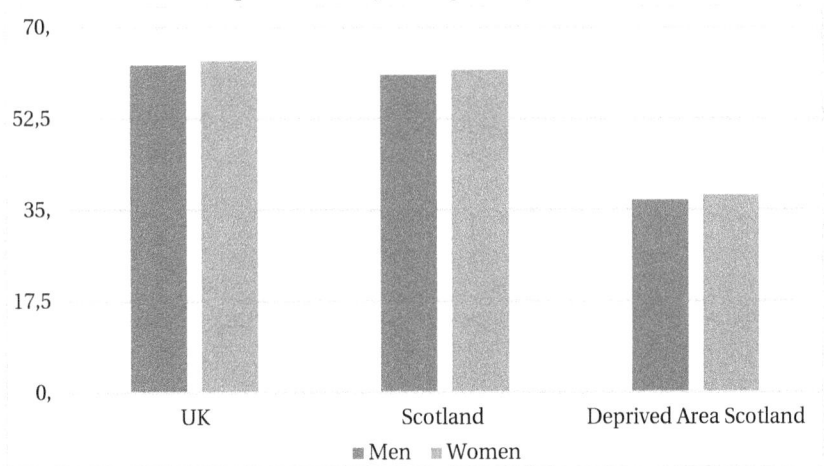

Data from: National Records of Scotland (2023) *Life Expectancy in Scotland 2019-2021.* Available at: https://www.nrscotland.gov.uk/files/statistics/life-expectancy-in-scotland/19-21/life-expectancy-19-21-report.pdf. Accessed: 20th August 2023.

The health of any individual in the UK owes much to their geographical and socio-economical position (BMA, 2022; Green, Filkin and Woods, 2021). In the past few years, the number of people waiting to see specialist consultants and registrars has increased significantly. Waiting times vary greatly between hospital trusts. This problem has been compounded by the coronavirus pandemic as the governments of all the home nations struggle to meet their waiting list targets. However, as will be discussed, these problems cannot solely be laid at the feet of those who run the country and the trusts.

Throughout the last 15 years, there have been many initiatives set up to try to promote better health, with prevention being better than cure. In 2007, the NHS Choices website was launched, followed in 2009 by the Change4Life campaign, FAST, the stroke campaign, and the NHS Health Check. These initiatives aimed to give individuals and their carers the tools and information necessary to make better health choices, to flag up potential issues such as heart disease or type 2 diabetes and to allow for early diagnosis of a stroke when time was critical. (Cohen, 2020). In this book, we will discuss, not only personal responsibility but will look at research which points to the health problems brought about by the government's austerity programme. The Lancet points out that in the UK, we have long-term health issues with "obesity, hypertension, chronic respiratory conditions, excess alcohol use and inactivity" (Green, Filkin and Woods, 2021, p. 1). The research literature we have utilised makes a note of COVID-19 and the pandemic, but it is too early for any long-term health effects to be analysed in great detail. Two of the participants' experiences occurred during the pandemic and the national lockdown and much reference is made to the psychological effects that had on the patients and their families. Data from my own experience alongside that of the health professionals makes very little reference to COVID-19 and therefore allows for comparison during and post-pandemic.

Scotland has an ageing population and as noted by the Scottish Government, "[b]y mid-2043, it is projected that 22.9% of the population will be of pensionable age, compared to 19.0% in mid-2018." (2021, p. 4). This brings problems and, as McLardy-Smith points out "[a] much more significant problem facing the NHS than waiting lists is the care of the elderly" (2022, p. 27). An ageing population increases the pressure on social care, the health service and family support (Elston et al. 2019; Leith and Sim, 2022). The pressure put on NHS Scotland may be due in part to the complex health needs of the elderly, we are already seeing an increase in the number of people diagnosed with dementia. It is predicted that the number of people requiring care will rise substantially in the following decades (Scottish Government, 2021). However, one must not overlook government budgets and the increased pressure caused by inflation.[6] Audit Scotland pointed out that "NHS services are not immune to

---

[6] At the time of writing this chapter, June 2023, UK inflation was running at 8.7%, down from a high of 11.2% in October 2022.

inflation and the NHS will face rising costs for everything from food to medicines." (2023, p. 12). The NHS is a costly service to run within the UK, with 40% of government expenditure being spent on providing health care. Much of that expenditure goes to treating those with multiple long-term conditions, around 70% of whom are situated in our elderly definition (McKee et al., 2021; Smith, 2023). Appleby and Gainsbury propose that planned expenditure for the two financial years 2022/23 and 2024/25 "will add a further £13.2billion in cash – although rising prices will cut this to around £2.4billion" (2022, p. 2). One question we ask is whether the NHS budget is being spent wisely and, if not, what changes can be made?

The data we collected points to iatrogenic disease/illness as a contributing factor in the deaths of two patients and the delay in treatment for a third. Coleman states that "iatrogenic illness needs to be taken seriously" (2022, p. 17). When considering the actions of the health professionals in their definition of iatrogenic injury Carvalho dos Santos and Ceolim put forward the following characterisation "whether right or wrong, justified or not, which originates harmful consequences for the patient's health" (2007, p. 809). Sirrs reminds us that "healthcare spaces such as hospitals have long been seen as sites of hazard" (2024, p. 2), noting that iatrogenic disease has been recognised for centuries. However, any preoccupation with patient safety is a relatively new one with iatrogenic harm now being viewed as a known medical hazard, one that is preventable (Gilmore et al., 2023; Sirrs, 2024). In 2000, the UK Department of Health published a report in response to high-profile scandals. The report looked into, amongst others, the Harold Shipman murders, the deaths of children undergoing heart surgery at Bristol Royal Infirmary as well as the unethical retention of organs at Alder's Hay Children's Hospital.[7] The report *An Organisation with a Memory* (AOWAM) "marks the key moment when 'patient safety' appeared

---

[7] **Harold Shipman** was a GP who, in 2000, was found guilty of the murder of 15 elderly patients and one count of fraud. His crimes were discovered after a family reported Shipman, when after the sudden death of their elderly mother, they discovered that her Will had been changed leaving Shipman as the sole beneficiary. Shipman was sentenced to life in prison but committed suicide soon after his sentencing. An inquiry later concluded that he may have committed 250 such murders.

**Bristol Royal Infirmary** saw, between 1991 and 1995, the deaths of between 30 and 35 children undergoing heart surgery that would probably have survived if operated on elsewhere in the NHS. The subsequent report highlighted flaws within the system from initial diagnosis to surgery to the set up between the operating theatres and ICU. There was seen to be a culture of silence and an *old boys' network*.

**Alder Hays Children's Hospital** was embroiled in a scandal in 1999 when it emerged that the hearts and other organs of 170 children who died at Bristol Royal Infirmary had been kept without family consent. The organs had been kept for research purposes.

on the policy agenda of the NHS" (Sirrs, 2024, p. 2), placing an emphasis on preventing iatrogenic harm within healthcare settings. Following the report, in 2001, the National Patient Safety Agency (NPSA) was established, acting as a patient safety learning centre for NHS staff and management. This was followed two years later by the National Reporting and Learning System (NRLS). The NRLS aimed to remove any barriers that impeded patients, and their families from making complaints when avoidable mistakes had been made. The intention was to remove the culture of silence and aimed to simplify the complaints procedure. Over the following years, the aforementioned patient safety departments have been strengthened. Patient safety was added as an NHS constitutional right in 2009 and the appointment of a Patient Safety Commissioner for England followed in 2022. The Scottish Government's Patient Safety Bill was added to the statute books in 2023. As the bill was passed the then Public Health Minister was quoted as saying:

> Our responsibility is to do all we can to make sure healthcare is made as safe as possible, and that in the future, when patients and families have concerns about the safety of their care, they do not have to struggle to make their voices heard. (Jenni Minto, cited in Scottish Government, 2023).

By analysing data from our participants, we will assess how effective the overhauling of the complaints system has been in Chapters Three and Five. As these chapters will demonstrate, our participants do not consider their voices to have been heard nor regard the complaints system to be an easy one to navigate.

One must consider the difference between iatrogenic incidents and those that are deemed negligent. Negligence can be described as a failure to use or provide an acceptable level of care therefore, as Sampath points out, "all harm that results from negligence is iatrogenic, not all iatrogenic injury is negligent" (2022, p. 736). Not all iatrogenic incidents stem from a failure to provide an acceptable level of care, these incidents can occur despite the best intentions of the staff. We must point out at this juncture that all hospitals have occurrences of iatrogeny and there are multiple reasons why this is the case:

- Tiredness caused by long working hours
- A lack of knowledge
- Pressure through being short-staffed

No matter the cause, Carvalho dos Santos and Ceolim point out that "[e]lderly patients are especially subject to the occurrence of iatrogenic events" (2007, p. 809). Further research highlights the increased risk elderly patients face from a range of causes: from adverse drug reactions to brain injuries caused by elder abuse and the dangers faced by dementia patients when transferred to and from various healthcare settings (Bugelli et al., 2023; Parker et al. 2021; Zazzara et al. 2021). Elder abuse is a worldwide hidden and under-reported problem, although it is estimated that 1 in 6 older adults have been abused in the past year (Bugelli et al., 2023, p. 2). Such abuse is usually perpetrated by a carer, be that in the home or in a health care setting.

There are many causes for this susceptibility, from complex health needs to an inability to self-advocate through dementia, or simply not wishing to question health professionals. Our (Dr Stead's and my own) parents held the medical profession in high esteem, this is something I have found, through talking to friends, is common among people in our parents' generation, the last generation to remember a time before the NHS. I have assumed that this reverence springs from a time when seeing a doctor was a luxury that one would only use when all other self-help routes had been exhausted. That a doctor had the knowledge and the ability to fix what other mere mortals could not and therefore they would never be questioned. However, Taylor has a simpler, and perhaps more disappointing, reason behind this susceptibility to iatrogenic disease "[a]ccepting of what the NHS does, or doesn't do to them, is wholly characteristic of today's elderly people and those low expectations without a doubt contribute to mediocre and inadequate responses throughout the system." (20 Feb, 2011). The plethora of bad news stories in the media may contribute to our low expectations. I suggest that we have a culture where one is dissuaded from complaining about a *free and accessible* service as we do not wish to be viewed as ungrateful, seen as criticising staff who, as the data will show, are working under stressful conditions.

Permpongkosol wrote that "the incidence of iatrogenic disease is between 3.4% and 33.9%" (2011, p. 8). He does not examine the reasons behind such a large range, but this may be due to how hospitals categorise and log such events as well as how many of these events are reported. What is known is that iatrogenic disease in the elderly has a greater impact than that of patients in younger age demographics (Permpongkosol, 2011; Carvalho dos Santos and Ceolim, 2007). This can be attributed to two factors "an absolute and percentage increase in the elderly population in parallel with an increased prevalence of iatrogenic pathology with age" (Permpongkosol, 2011, p. 78). It is problematic to ratify, with any certainty, Coleman's view that through iatrogenic disease, "doctors and health care workers are one of the three top causes of death" (2022, p. 17). One could not confirm such an assertion when hospitals have such different ways of classifying such incidents. We aim to examine the reasons behind the vulnerability of the elderly to iatrogeny and to consider ways in which this could be reduced or, at the very least, have a lesser detrimental health impact. We also look into incidences of iatrogenic harm suffered by NHS Scotland staff, both mental and physical.

## The Hospital

The Queen Elizabeth University Hospital (QEUH) is a 1,677-bed acute hospital located in Govan, in the south-west of Glasgow, Scotland. The hospital was built on the site of the former Southern General Hospital and opened at the end of April 2015. It was built to replace/relocate five Glasgow hospitals:

- The Western Infirmary
- The Victoria Infirmary
- The Southern General Hospital
- The Queen Mother Maternity Hospital
- The Royal Hospital for Sick Children, Yorkhill

I was interested to find out the rationale behind the closing of the aforementioned hospitals and the decision to locate the QEUH on the Southern General site. I was unable to gain any information from relevant governmental bodies. I can only surmise that as the Victoria Infirmary was a Victorian building and the other four hospitals were built in the 1960s and 1970s, their general upkeep was proving costly. The land the hospitals were situated on was prime for development. Following closure, the Victoria, Western, Queen Mother and Southern General hospitals were all, or are in the process of being, demolished. The Southern General site now, as mentioned, houses the QEUH. The Western Infirmary, as part of its original covenant, was given to Glasgow University. The university has used some of the 14-acre site for university state-of-the-art research hubs, whilst a proportion has been sold for commercial development. A section of the Victoria Infirmary plot is the site of a new hospital, the New Victoria Hospital. This hospital is an outpatient clinic and diagnostic hub, as well as a minor injury unit. The other section of land was sold to a private house-building company. The Royal Hospital for Sick Children, Yorkhill, has also been re-commissioned as an outpatient diagnostic unit. At present, I could not find information on the plans for the Queen Mother site, and demolition is due to be completed by autumn 2024.

I sent the following email to the NHSGGC requesting information on the rationale behind closing the aforementioned hospitals and the building of the QEUH. The request was made under the Freedom of Information Act 2005 (FOI):

Under the Freedom of Information Act, I would like to request the following information:

1. Any documents that contain the rationale for closing the Western Infirmary, the Victoria Infirmary, the Southern General Hospital, The Queen Mother Maternity Hospital and the Royal Hospital for Sick Children and relocating all services to a new hospital on the site of the old Southern General.
2. The average ambulance response time/ waiting time outside hospitals for the calendar year 2022 and in the 3 years prior to and after this change.
3. The average waiting time for an A&E bed for the calendar 2022 and in the 3 years prior to and after this change

Please contact me if you need me to clarify my request, at ********* or 0**********

Dr Yvonne Bennett

Despite section 10 of the Freedom of Information Act stating that a reply to a request must be received no later than 20 working days following the date of receipt of the request, I have yet to receive a response. As part of my research for this book I sent five different FOI requests to five different NHS Scotland departments with the following results: three failed to respond, despite follow up emails, a fourth replied that it was not in the public interest and the fifth responded, within five days, with the information I had requested. I mentioned this to my daughter in law, she had once worked for the Scottish Government, and one part of her job was answering FOIs. She informed me that I had to be extremely precise in the wording of my request as to do otherwise would mean a rejection of the request. This was a loophole used to stop information from being given out that the government may not want to be released. As a result, I have no official answers to the following questions:

1. the number of complaints NHS Scotland has received every year for the last 3 calendar years.

2. Of those complaints received each year, the number that are upheld by a) the NHS and b) the Ombudsman.

3. Of those complaints received each year, the number that that are dismissed.

4. The number of complaints the Scottish Ambulance Service has received every year for the last 3 calendar years.

5. Of those complaints received each year, the number that are upheld by a) the NHS and b) the Ombudsman.

6. Of those complaints received each year, the number that are dismissed.

I do however have data referring to the number of student nurses within NHS Scotland from application to graduation. This data will be analysed in reference to one of the RCN's proposed solutions to assist with nurse recruitment and the alleviation of unsafe staffing levels.

The QEUH comprises a 1,109-bed adult hospital, a 256-bed children's hospital and two major Emergency Departments: one for adults and one for children. The QEUH is not without its controversies and long-term problems. Since its opening, there have been inquiries into the deaths of two children, with the mainstream media reporting that "[t]oxic dust from a demolition site next to Scotland's flagship hospital caused water supply contamination which led to deadly infections in patients." (Robertson and Rodgers, 2023). The QEUH was under construction whilst the old Southern General Hospital was being demolished. You also cannot help but notice the QEUH's proximity to a sizeable sewage treatment plant when the wind is blowing in its direction.

Following an outbreak of bacterial infections in 2017, which included 51 children receiving treatment for blood cancer, a series of independent investigations and inquiries concluded that the hospital's water supply was contaminated before its opening in 2015. The Scottish Hospitals' Inquiry went as far as to state:

> [f]luctuations in the water temperature experienced since the opening of the hospital were also a likely contributing factor; and that fungus in the water system was likely due to the dust levels around the site during construction and demolitions.... To understand where the bacteria was located within the water supply, samples were taken from all parts of the water system. Results showed that all floors had some contamination, indicating that the problem was widespread. (Robertson and Rodgers, 2023).

Despite findings by a further inquiry in 2019 by the NHS body, Health Facilities Scotland, which appeared to agree with other inquiries, a Greater Glasgow Health Board spokesman was quoted in the media as saying the reports "have not been analysed or investigated by the inquiry nor have they been proved to be factually correct." (Robertson and Rodgers, 2023). Contaminated water was not the only source of bacteria found during investigations into the cause of the deaths of the young patients:

> the presence of cockroaches, fungal odour, room not ventilated, water ingress and dried algae present on the floor. Further checks on the child cancer ward, 2A, discovered 'thick black and yellow grime was visible in the drains'. The documents state that two out of three patient infections matched swabs taken from the drains which revealed bacteria. The

health board agreed to close the ward for refurbishment after pressure from senior medics. (Robertson and Rodgers, 2023).

The refurbishment of the QEUH was to take over three years to complete at a cost of around £11 million. Yet despite solving many of the problems, a new filtration water system and new ventilation shafts to name but a few, the problem with the stench of sewage remains, something I can personally attest to. At the time of writing this book, two new problems have blighted the hospital; unsafe cladding and the use of reinforced autoclaved aerated concrete (Raac) have been identified in some of the older buildings on the campus.[8]

## Method

For this research, we used an ethnographic methodology. Along with video content and comments from TikTok, data was gathered utilising semi-structured interviews. We have included my own story in the research as not only was it the catalyst that ignited this body of work, but I was mindful of Katz-Rothman's (2007) work in which she wrote of how, as academics, we have been encouraged to remove our voice from our research in the interest of supposed objectivity. For all researchers, "there is a degree of personal investment in choosing the area of research" (Hervieu-Léger 2000, p. 13). With this in mind, I am of the opinion that total objectivity is almost impossible to achieve and as such, I wanted my subjective experiences to be noted. Putnam and Banghart noted that as researchers bring a degree of bias to the research field and subsequent analysis, "value free data or complete neutrality does not exist in interpretive work" (2017, p. 7). As researchers, we must tread a line between reflecting everything that comes before us and keeping it at a distance, a balance between striking a relationship with the participants and remaining detached. With this in mind, any preconceived values and biases must become a part of the data under analysis. Understanding why one has chosen the research topic and the possibility of pre-held conceptions must be scrutinised alongside the data to ensure an in-depth analysis.

One consequence of employing an ethnographic framework is that we had, just by our presence, an effect on the participants. We are outsiders and, as such, cannot help but alter the dynamic. When carrying out interviews we entered their social sphere as researchers yet brought our history and our own experiences. Dr Stead and I belong to the *sandwich generation* and that was an

---

[8] The cladding used on the outside of the atrium of the QEUH is not fire retardant and is being replaced at a cost of £33 million. Raac is a lightweight concrete that has been widely used throughout Europe since the 1950s. It has since been found to have a life span of around 30 years and can fail and collapse at any time, with no prior warning. Many public buildings in the UK are affected by this with schools being forced to close.

aspect of our lives we had in common with three of the participants.[9] It was this facet of our identities that helped us build a rapport with these contributors. With any ethnographic study it is difficult to disconnect the researcher from the researched, using life stories makes the study a joint venture, with the researcher becoming the channel through which the story is passed to a wider audience (Maines, Pierce and Laslett, 2008). As my own experience with NHS Scotland was the stimulus that began this research, I became both a participant and researcher; therefore, the first data collected was my own. The need to understand and analyse my story is rooted in our decision to utilise a constructivist approach to data analysis. A full depth analysis of the approach used will be examined fully in a subsequent chapter. This will look at ethical considerations alongside our rationale behind the methodology used.

How we have situated the personal stories that form the foundation of the book has been done so in a deliberate manner. The details chosen for inclusion attempt a balance between narrative necessity and examples of the themes that are examined. Maines, Pierce and Laslett noted the importance of participants and researchers "speaking the same language" (2008, p. 114); therefore, it was important that we used the participant's own words to describe their parent, their experiences, and their trauma. This also contributed to us situating the stories as a standalone chapter as it ensures that the participants could see their stories without them being obscured by academic language.

It was important to remove the personal stories of the elderly, the stories of who these individuals were, and what they meant to their families, from the traumatic experiences that are a part of the book's data. People are shaped by their experiences and backgrounds but are "never reducible to them" (Maines, Pierce and Laslett, 2008, p. 181). We have done so using a precise at the beginning of Chapter Two. It was important to the families that we kept their names, that they were recognisable by those who knew and loved them. However, the medical staff who came forward have been given a cloak of anonymity, and their names have been changed. They have also been afforded the right to see the transcripts of their interviews. This has allowed them to clarify certain aspects and to have any identifying parts removed. We also wanted to give a clear voice to all the participants' experiences, to draw a well-defined line between their stories and analytical data. We are more than just a statistic.

---

[9] The sandwich generation is a term used to define adults, around the ages of 40-60 years who care for elderly parents as well as raising and assisting their own children. This assistance has stretched because, as the 2021 Census for England and Wales revealed, "About 30% of 25- to 29-year-olds now live with their parents, and more than one in 10 (11.6%) adult children aged 30 to 34 – up from 8.6% in 2011." (Booth and Goodier, 2023).

Cohen pointed out that "the challenges that the fledgling NHS faced were enormous and decisions made in these early years.... were to shape NHS treatment and policy for decades to come" (2020, p. 25). Advances in medical science meant that new illnesses were discovered along with new treatments. Bevan's vision was that as people became healthier the cost to the NHS would decline as it would be needed less. Sadly, the opposite happened as people made more and more demands on it. Demands that are not always realistic. The purpose of this book is to shed light on the ways that NHS Scotland has let down its elderly and how our complacent use of our proud institution is aiding in its downfall.

# List of Abbreviations

| | |
|---|---|
| **A&E** | Accident and Emergency |
| **AOWAM** | An Organisation with a Memory |
| **BMT** | Bone Marrow Transplant |
| **COPD** | Chronic Obstructive Pulmonary Disease |
| **CPR** | Cardiopulmonary Resuscitation |
| **DNR** | Do Not Resuscitate |
| **ESW** | Emergency Service Workers |
| **F&E** | Facilities and Estates |
| **FOI** | Freedom of Information Act |
| **FPC** | Free Personal Care |
| **FPNC** | Free Personal Nursing Care |
| **GMC** | General Medical Council |
| **GP** | General Practitioner |
| **HESA** | Higher Education Statistics Agency |
| **HIS** | Healthcare Improvement Scotland |
| **HOIC** | The History of Infection Control |
| **ICD** | Infection Control Doctor |
| **ICU** | Intensive Care Unit |
| **IF** | In-patient fall |
| **IRH** | Inverclyde Royal Hospital |
| **IV** | Intravenous |
| **LDP** | Local Delivery Plan |
| **MSP** | Member of Scottish Parliament |
| **NHS** | National Health Service |
| **NHSGGC** | National Health Service Greater Glasgow and Clyde Health Board |
| **NICE** | National Institute for Care Excellence |
| **NPSA** | National Patient Safety Agency |
| **NRLS** | National Reporting and learning System |
| **PCC** | Patient Centred Care |
| **QEUH** | Queen Elizabeth University Hospital |
| **Raac** | Reinforced autoclaved aerated concrete |
| **RAH** | Royal Alexandra Hospital |
| **RCN** | Royal College of Nursing |
| **RGN** | Registered General Nurse |
| **SAS** | Scottish Ambulance Service |
| **SNP** | Scottish National Party |
| **STV** | Scottish Television |
| **YYF** | Ysbyty Ystrad Fawr (Hospital) |

# Chapter One

# Methodology and Ethical Considerations

## Christina Stead

The research reported in this book arose from a social media post made by Dr Yvonne Bennett on Thursday 11th August 2022.[1] A video published on TikTok, telling the story of her mother's hospitalisation as an in-patient at the QEUH, went viral and attracted nearly 300,000 views. When posting, there had been no intention to gather data for a research publication, however, given the level and nature of responses, it quickly became clear that there was a wider story worth researching. In this chapter, we explain the methodology and research methods adopted and then discuss the ethical considerations that arose as we developed the project.

The book draws on data collected via qualitative research in an ethnographic framework. A range of different methods of data collection was used, including interviews, textual analysis and statistical data. Katz-Rothman (2007) proposes that the written word is narration, recounted by the author. Remove the author from the text and the account becomes passive. Initially, we considered taking an autobiographical approach but, although this would have enabled us to situate ourselves within the research, it would have placed our personal stories at the centre (Stanley 1993). This was not a position that we wished to occupy because the research tells more than our own stories.

Epistemologically, we take a constructivist position that knowledge can be gained inductively from interacting with people and gathering material on their lived subjective experiences. Within this framework, there is an explicit acknowledgement of the relationship between the researcher and the individual telling the story. We take a relativist ontology in that, as human beings, we each construct our subjective version of 'reality', relative to our individual experiences and influences. As no two humans will share identical thoughts, there cannot, therefore, be a single worldview. *Truth* or *fact* for one person will not be the same for another, because both constructs arise from individual perceptions.

The subject matter of this book encompasses highly sensitive personal stories, including the deaths of three much-loved parents and the subsequent

---

[1] See: https://www.tiktok.com/@yvonnecooks6/video/7130366122288794885?is_from_webapp=1&sender_device=pc&web_id=7290897856394708512

grief felt by family members, as well as sometimes harrowing narratives of difficult working lives within the Scottish health service. These are all factors that, inevitably, have affected the collection and interpretation of the data but are consistent with this type of qualitative research (Oakley, 1981; Harraway, 1988). As noted in the Introduction, it is possible to trace multiple subjectivities within this study, arising from the participants, from us as researchers/ participants, and from the nature of the topic, the experience of elderly care in the particular setting of Glasgow. The role of reflexivity, or critical self-reflection, is important (Savickas, 2011; Peavy, 1992; Richardson, 1997) because it equips human beings to look at the present through the lens of the past and to re/negotiate realities. It also provides a mechanism for paying close attention to the contextual situation of the narrative. We return to reflexivity later in the chapter.

Given our epistemological position and the subject matter of the research, we used narrative methods to gather data. The use of narrative/storytelling is a widely accepted form of qualitative research and can offer a bridge between an individual and the prevailing cultural system, for, as Wright Mills (1959) noted, a narrative can help its teller to link the personal to the public. This is crucial to the current study, concerned as it is with the individual stories behind NHS headlines and data. In responding to the TikTok post, participants had already engaged with the narrative, in that they had started to offer their stories. By following up with interviews, we were extending and deepening the narrative process. Within this, we recognized that we were not seeking or gaining factual objectivity. As Plummer suggests, "the narrative of a life is not *the* life" (2001, p.185) because it is a representation that reflects subjectivity and temporality and is, therefore, likely to change.

The book draws on ethnographic data gathered from four interviews as well as Dr Bennett's own story. The interviews were held with people who had contacted Dr Bennett after viewing her TikTok post. The table below summarises the response to the post. She received a mixture of direct, private messaging and public comment, with a clear split between genders. The majority of men made political comments, often pro- or anti-SNP or Brexit. Most of the women who publicly commented had their own stories to tell and wanted to offer sympathy or empathy. All the private messages came from women, again offering sympathy, empathy and/or stories of personal experiences. Like Dr Bennett, some were the relatives of patients, whilst others were employed in different parts of the health services; they shared a desire for their narratives to enter the public domain, albeit with appropriate anonymity for the employees to protect their working lives.[2]

**Figure 1.1** Responses to Yvonne Bennett's TikTok Post of 12th August 2022.

| | |
|---|---|
| Number of views | 299,300 |
| Number of likes | 19,400 |
| Number of comments | 2610 |
| Number of shares | 770 |
| Saved to favourites | 791 |
| Number of private messages | 12 |
| | Number of staff 6 (4 nurses, 1 paramedic, 1 care home employee)<br>Number of family stories 6 |
| Agreed to interview | 10 |
| Signed consent forms and proceeded to interview | 4 (1 nurse, 1 paramedic, 2 family stories) |

Several people who initially agreed to be interviewed withdrew from the project because they could not afford to compromise their working situations. Before the four interviews went ahead, each participant received a summary sheet explaining the aims of the project and then signed a consent form.[3] We explained that we were interested in experiences of elderly care at the QEUH and would be happy to meet participants in person or online. As we did not personally know any of the participants before this project, it was important to establish rapport so that they would feel comfortable talking to us. We were cognizant of the need to establish trust and transparency in the research relationship. As a participant, Dr Bennett was conscious that her role would be "characterised as that of dual identity" (Reed-Dannahay 1997, p. 3). She was both researcher and participant, both insider and outsider (Blumer 1969; Stanley 1993). I (Christina Stead) was not a participant in the sense of being interviewed for the project, however, I also occupy that insider-outsider territory as part of my role in data collection, analysis and writing up the

---

[2] Roseanne had already taken her story to news outlets and had appeared on national television in Scotland.

[3] We have included a copy of the information sheet in an appendix. We have not included the consent forms as they contain personal information.

research. Both these circumstances correlated with the principle of symbolic interactionism and the proposal that all individuals self-identify through social interaction, taking on roles depending on the social situation (Shibutani, 1970). We were aware, however, that:

> in social research, the distribution of power is not always tilted in favour of the researcher; oftentimes the participants command greater power over the research process: its progression as well as the amount and quality of data the ethnographer has access to. (Mapedzahama and Dune 2017, p.5).

Participants had contacted us in response to Dr Bennett's story because they wanted to tell us (and, in the case of those who agreed to be interviewed, for us to retell) their stories. It seems clear that the TikTok post had stimulated some recognition of shared experience based around the QEUH, however, it was important to give space for the participants to share their individual stories. We, therefore, used semi-structured interviews because we sought narratives that were meaningful to them: our questions were deliberately broad to give space for the stories to be told. Congruent with an ethnographic approach, it was important to understand when to talk and when to be silent; at all times, our primary responsibility was to listen to our participants because we wanted our work to illuminate and contribute to the overall understanding of the care of the elderly in the QEUH/NHS Scotland. All this was also ontologically consistent with qualitative and interpretive research (Holloway and Jefferson, 2013).

In their responses on TikTok, our participants had already begun to share stories about the broader lives, hospital care and deaths of their relatives, or about their workplace experiences, hence, it made sense to adopt narrative research methods. One key reason for this choice was that narrative offers a bridge between the individual and the prevailing cultural system, linking, as Wright Mills (1959) noted, the personal to the public. In exploring individual stories, we looked at the complexity, contradiction and constraints of everyday life (Hodkinson and Hodkinson, 2001). Whilst the use of narrative as a research method is well-established, it is a complex field that can encompass different elements and comes with a somewhat contested definition (Riessman, 2008; Speedy, 2008; Horsdal, 2012; Andrews et al., 2013).

For this book, we focus on the element of *story*, drawn from social media interactions and subsequent interviews. This was because individuals make sense of their world through stories (Goffman 1959). We had to set clear parameters for the project, including boundaries and ethical considerations, as later discussed. We also had to be mindful of what Squire (2013) refers to as the over-interpretation of data. Whilst the use of interviews may represent a conservative approach to research methods, we judged that interviews offered the best opportunity to secure participation and, to facilitate this further, we offered a choice of face-to-face or online interactions to suit each participant's preference. Though initially focused on narratives around care, particularly of the elderly, the research also touched on what Denzin and Lincoln describe as "the constraints of everyday life" (2011, p.5) because the stories shared by each participant are also part of a wider and coherent life story.

Storytelling involving participant memories raises complex issues regarding time and chronology (Josselson, 2009, 2011). Narratives are necessarily a re-presentation of events drawn from autobiographical memory, which is described as the *glue* in narrative meaning-making (Fivush, 2019, p.2). Participants spoke to us about sensitive, emotional issues, and this impacted the structure of their narratives. For example, when Tracy told her father's story, the sequencing of the events was unclear at times and could be difficult to follow. In the interview, we sought clarification where we could but did not want to interrupt the flow of the narrative unnecessarily. The literature indicates that stories may vary depending on the point at which listening takes place (Andrews et al., 2013) and that narrative stories can be big or small (Savickas, 2011; Phoenix, 2013). Big stories are narratives such as life histories, whereas small stories are gleaned from everyday encounters. This research encompassed both types, particularly in the cases of Roseanne and Tracy, because they wanted to tell us about the lives of, respectively, their mother and father and to emphasise that they were people who had embraced life in all its messy complexities before they became mortality statistics. Sam and Jordan recounted episodes in their professional lives, largely everyday encounters if the description above is used, but connected to the wider context of the management of the health service.

The interviews with Roseanne, Tracy (accompanied by her daughter, Jamie-Lee) and Jordan were held in person in Glasgow, with both researchers in attendance. Yvonne Bennett interviewed Sam alone, during a visit to Scotland to see family. The in-person interviews were held in venues suggested by the participants: the majority chose busy cafes, so the recordings include the noises of everyday life going on around us. This was especially poignant given the emotional impact of some of the testimony.

We recorded each interview as unobtrusively as possible on a mobile phone and then transcribed the material manually; this helped us to immerse ourselves in the materials that we had generated. For *Jordan* and *Sam*, who both worked within the health services, we adopted gender-neutral aliases and they/them pronouns to anonymise the data and protect their identities. The other participants were offered anonymity or the opportunity to be identified via the use of their real names. In social research, the use of pseudonyms is standard because of the risks that might arise from identification, but Tracy and

Roseanne wanted their stories to be recognisable, hence, we have used their full names. There is a growing recognition that it is not harmful to use real names and instead explicitly record input from a participant, as long as the implications are understood. Whilst not necessarily the safest or most comfortable approach to take, it can be the most respectful (Tillman, 2015). As already noted, Roseanne had been sharing her mother's story widely to publicise her concerns. She and Tracy were also happy to provide photographs and other family memorabilia for reproduction in the book.

## Reflexivity

It was important to be reflexive as we collected and analysed the data. This helped to guard against the risk that our data, particularly Dr Bennett's, would take too prominent a position within the project, chiming with Adjepong's view that "[r]eflexivity addresses the assumptions that the researcher might take with them into the field, examines how their presence shaped the social setting and consequently avoids producing a flawed sociology" (2017, p.31). For Etherington, reflexivity operates well alongside a constructivist ontology. She suggests that combining the two can help the researcher "avoid accusations of solipsism, self-indulgence, navel gazing or narcissism" (2004, p. 31).

Social media sites provide opportunities for users to put private expressions of feeling in the public domain. As demonstrated by Dr Bennett's reflections below, the stimuli are not always clear and, indeed, are part of a continually shifting psychological and emotional landscape, particularly at times of distress such as serious family illness. Whether generating or responding to content, the decision to comment in a public space may provide emotional relief or the opportunity to connect with a community of users with similar experiences (Selman et al., 2021). In the spirit of critical self-reflection, Yvonne Bennett writes:

> I was using digital storytelling to produce and project my message. Online disinhibition... was it a game? I would not have stood in the car park and shared my traumatic experience with complete strangers who were physically there so why did I speak to a multiplicity of online strangers? Was it to move, or complete, the narrative? To preserve the memory? To make it available to revisit? By telling my story, I was not only sharing my vulnerability, but I was, perhaps, hoping to find a degree of understanding from both myself, and a multitude of keyboard strangers. Did using TikTok make me feel respected, listened to, and validated? The comments were, on the whole, positive, and empathetic. There were, however, some distressing comments from trolls. Despite pretending that these do not matter and deleting/blocking the account

holders, these messages have a profoundly upsetting effect. Storytelling is a powerful and healing way to cope with trauma and stress. It can help you express, reframe, and connect with your experiences, feelings, and insights. (Yvonne Bennett, 2023).

## Ethical Considerations

The ethics inherent in this project were complex. In addition to standard considerations attached to qualitative research, the participant narratives encompassed stories of death, alleged medical negligence, unsafe workplace practices and the consequences of whistleblowing. It was crucially important to draw boundaries around what it was acceptable and proper to discuss in this book and what fell outside our remit. In the interviews, the participants (understandably) drew no such boundaries and shared the information that was important to them; consequently, the transcripts contain material that is not appropriate to analyse except in the broadest terms. This includes Roseanne, Tracy, and Jamie-Lee's comments on the specific circumstances around their respective relative's death. In addition to their empathetic responses to Dr Bennett's TikTok post, it is possible that participants had other motives for speaking to us, including the potential for catharsis, altruism (Alexander, 2013) or simply wider publicity.

As with any research on a sensitive topic, the potential for harm to participants had to be considered. We are independent researchers (and thus did not have to seek ethical approval from a committee) but were mindful of good practice and had experience in navigating challenging ethical landscapes from previous ethnographic (Bennett, 2020) and biographical (Stead, 2020) projects. Formal ethics, such as those handed down from a committee, had the potential to be legalistic and possibly also paternalistic (Pascoe Leahy, 2022); such an approach would not have suited this project where any difficulties would have needed to be negotiated in situ. At all times, we were mindful of the obligation to minimise possible harm to the participants, however, we took the view that each person was capable of setting their parameters concerning the disclosure of information. As researchers, we were acutely aware of the delicacy of the subject matter and sought to treat our participants with respect and care. In addition to summary information on the nature, purpose and potential risks of the research process, each participant was also made aware that they could withdraw from the process at any point. They were then asked to give informed consent and to sign the appropriate documentation. The interviews were recorded between November 2022 and January 2023. Jordan and Sam's narratives reflect their workplace situations at the time of the interview as well as covering some previous events. It should be noted that Sam has now left their job.

The notion of informed consent was problematic because, whilst information on the structure and purpose of the project could readily be provided for the participants, it was more difficult to explain what would happen to their narratives during the analytical part of the research process. This is particularly relevant to the detailed medical information shared by Rosanne and Tracy that could not be analysed in the book, however, there is also a more general issue, in that it is rarely possible to use all the material provided by a participant, so selection has to be made by the researchers. Whilst we were cautious of claiming to *give voice* to our participants when the material has been selected and interpreted by us as part of the analytical process, feedback from the participants indicates that they saw this as a platform from which their voices could be heard.

Our guiding principles in analysing the material from the transcripts were integrity and trustworthiness (Riessman, 2008). The interviews generated rich data which we supplemented with literature and statistical data that could help to explain what was happening at the QEUH, thereby connecting the personal to the public and political. Whilst our research is drawn from the narratives of a small sample of participants, those stories give illumination to the broader picture of elderly care in the hospital. For Yvonne Bennett, who is both author and participant, analysis of the situation in QEUH began as she sought to make sense of her mother's situation. The interviewing and analytical processes were intertwined as we began mentally sifting and reviewing the material in situ, as recognised by Merrill and West (2009) and Andrews et al. (2013). Once we had produced the transcripts, key themes were identified and selected via a proforma approach developed by Merrill and West (2009). We considered using a basic coding system based on keywords, however quickly realised that this was a reductive process that risked diluting the nuance and context of the participants 'stories and did not lend itself to interpretive analysis.

The next step was to write chapters based on the themes identified in the proformas and draw on pertinent literature. An ethical issue was raised as a result of this, namely the level of involvement that should be offered to the participants at this point. Whilst there is precedent for including participants in the analytical phase of research (Tilmann, 2015), our view was that it was not appropriate in either practical or logistical terms. We had only requested participation in interviews and could not realistically have asked for input into the academic analysis as that would have changed the character and outcome of the project. That is not to say that there was not the capacity for an interesting methodological contribution through the further involvement of participants.

We were also aware that, as researchers, we would have judgements made about us. Understanding this concept was vital for data analysis as we endeavoured to be both objective and subjective. Chang interestingly described the dynamic between objectivity and subjectivity as a "tug of war" (2008, p. 45), a conflict that shapes debate surrounding social research that is situated within an ethnographic framework. We consciously chose to place our own "personal and subjective interpretation into the research process" (Chang 2008, p. 45). As described above, our interviews were transcribed, so the information is there in black and white, however, the conversations before and after taping also yielded rich data. Writing this up was reliant on memory and memory is selective, subjective, and open to question (Stanley 1993). Ethnography requires external, broad-based data as a measure to both strengthen and validate the internal subjective data (Chang 2008). We have, therefore, used external data from the Scottish government and health services to corroborate the material drawn from interviews and social media sources.

### "Leaving the research"

We were keen that participants should continue to feel connected to the research after they had been interviewed, however, conscious of individual preferences and time constraints, we did not wish to be prescriptive as to what form this might take. Administrative protocols were followed, in that after the interviews had been completed, and in accordance with the information on the consent forms, the participants were offered the opportunity to check their transcripts. Only Jordan and Sam took this up, probably reflecting a need to check that their jobs would not be compromised. We also shared the material included in Chapter Two (Our Stories) and asked if any revisions should be made. Tracy and Roseanne were asked to provide photographs if they wished, however, this could not apply to the others because of the need for anonymity. The iterative nature of the analysis was such that it was not possible to give updates of findings as is suggested as good practice in guidelines from the NHS Health Research Authority (2023). Dr Bennett has, however, maintained an online *open door* and, whilst she has received a small number of messages, regular communication has not been forthcoming. This is not surprising, given the pressures and shifting priorities of daily life: indeed, the stories in this book are not static and it was also important to be reflexive as we collected and analysed the data. This helped to guard against the risk that our data, particularly Dr Bennett's, would take too prominent a position within the project, chiming with Adjepong's view that "[r]eflexivity addresses the assumptions that the researcher might take with them into the field, examines how their presence shaped the social setting and consequently avoids producing a flawed sociology" (2017, p.31). For Etherington (2004), reflexivity operates well alongside a constructivist ontology. She suggests that combining the two can help the researcher avoid being accused of narcissistic or self-indulgent behaviours.

Our approach to maintaining connections with research participants after their interviews was considerate of individual preferences and time constraints. Our commitment to reflexivity, aligned with the principles of Adjepong (2017) and Etherington (2004), guided us in avoiding potential pitfalls and maintaining a balanced and ethical research approach. As the book neared completion, Dr Bennett contacted each participant to ask for feedback on the process. Specifically, they were asked why they had chosen to be interviewed and how they now felt, a year after. Participants will be offered copies of the book, so publication may provide an impetus for further communication with the authors in due course.

# Chapter Two

# **Our Stories**

Yvonne Bennett

We have chosen to use storytelling as a way of locating the data we analysed. Page wrote "[s]tories remain a pervasive genre that people use to make sense of themselves and the surrounding world." (2018, p. 1). This chapter will let the reader get to know the participants as it focuses attention on a much-loved family member or, in the case of the staff members, gives an insight into the struggles and frustrations they experience working for NHS Scotland. The following chapters are not giving a subjective history of the COVID-19 pandemic but aim to allow the reader to "reflect on and explore the individuals' place in collective events" (Maines, Pierce and Laslett, 2008, p. 43). These are our stories.

## The Participants

### Helen (Ella) Nimmo: 18/3/1933 – 29/3/2023

Our mum was seven months pregnant with me when my brother, Billy, drowned just three weeks before his sixth birthday. This has, and always will have, an impact on my life despite my never knowing him. Some of my earliest memories are of visiting his grave with my parents and Graeme, my younger brother. To this day I can see the tap where my mum and dad changed the water for the flowers and the bin beside it filled with dead flowers and cigarette butts.

Billy named both of us surviving siblings, even though he never met us. He wanted the new baby to be named Yvonne if a girl, and Graeme, if a boy, as these were the names of his closest friends at school. We carry his legacy with us. Few people know of Billy, as it is difficult to mention him without receiving, either an embarrassed silence or excessive sympathy, neither of which I feel is appropriate. I carry no personal grief, although the sorrow I felt for my parents is enormous.

What Graeme and I didn't know was that when Billy was three years old my parents suffered the tragedy of a stillbirth, another son lost. Our mum only told me of his death when Graeme and his wife were expecting their first child, our parent's first grandchild. Our mum experienced so much loss at a time when such tragedies were never discussed. She never saw the baby; she never knew what happened to him. Years later my daughter, then twelve or thirteen years of age, gave our dad a memory book for Christmas. He had to fill it out and give it back to her. In it he wrote that the baby was to have been called Gordon, he had a name. Following our dad's death in 2022 and mum's accident, it was clear that she would need care for the rest of her life and never return home, the house had to be sold. In clearing it Graeme found a box with *important* papers in it. There he found a receipt for an undertaker for Gordon's burial. He has a grave, something my mum never knew. Sadly, as was the usual occurrence in the 1950s, Gordon was buried with a stranger and although the cemetery confirmed that he was indeed buried on 21st July 1959, they have no record of who he was interned with. There is a memorial at the cemetery to all the 'lost' babies who are buried there, a memorial Graeme and I will visit.

Our mum was more than just the tragic experiences that marred her life. A farmer's daughter who hated to cook, the middle child of five with two older brothers and two younger sisters. The possessor of a dry sense of humour and a multitude of funny sayings that would stop you in your tracks. A young mum born and raised in rural East Lothian, Scotland but who moved hundreds of miles west to the industrial shipbuilding town of Greenock to be a policeman's wife. A woman who worked for *pin money* as a Provie wuman.[1,2] A woman who raised two children, eight grandchildren and welcomed into the world two great-granddaughters. A woman who was married for 67 years but was more than just Sandy's wife. A woman that we all miss dreadfully.

---

[1] Pin money is the term used for money earned by women through part-time employment. This money helped with household finances or, if lucky, could be used for treats.

[2] The Provie wumen is a colloquial term for a Provident agent working for Provident Personal Credit. Provident are different to most other personal loan lenders, as self-employed agents they visit clients in their own homes. In the 1970s and 80s, when my mum was an agent, most loans came in the form of cheques that local stores would accept. The repayments would be made weekly with agents, such as my mum, visiting the clients at home to collect an agreed amount. As agents live and work within the community that they serve, it means that they have a greater understanding of the area and the issues that the community faces. Our mum remained friends with many of her clients.

Image 2.1 Sandy and Ella Nimmo 26/12/2018.[3]

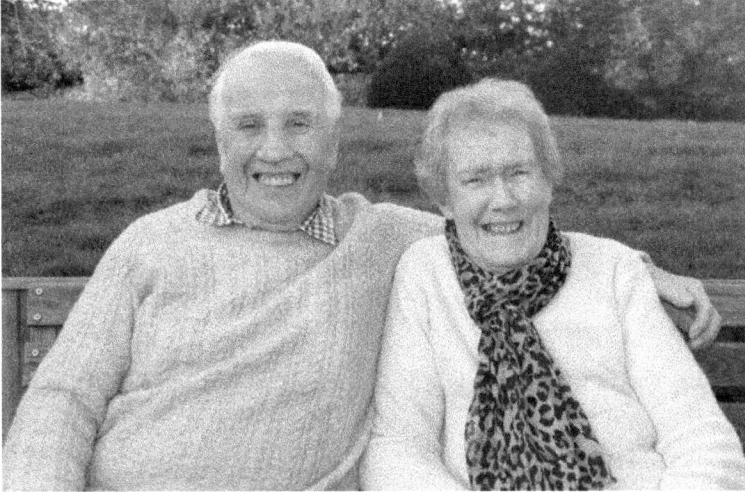

## Jean Wingate: 16/10/1944 – 3/11/2020

Our mum was the matriarch of the family, raising nine children as a single mum, a widow. She was the centre of the family, the cornerstone, and everything revolved around her. This is her story; this is who she was.

Our mum and dad were married when mum was 19 years old, becoming a mum within the year. Our dad was at Ibrox Stadium on the day of their wedding watching Glasgow Rangers Football Club, I don't know who they were playing or the result.[4] What I do know, however, is that Dad's best man had to have an announcement made over the tannoy to get him to his wedding on time.[5][6]

Our mum had eleven children, nine of whom survived into adulthood. She experienced tragedy, having one daughter, Jean, stillborn and a son, Thomas, who died when he was only three months old. As was common in those days the hospital dealt with the burial arrangements for Jean and we do not know where she was laid to rest. Thomas was buried with my grandparents. Both children are named on mum's tombstone. At 39 years of age, our mum was

---

[3] All photos belong to the families who agreed to participate in this research and have been used with their permission.

[4] Ibrox Stadium is the home ground of Glasgow Rangers FC. The stadium is an iconic Glasgow landmark in the Govan area of Glasgow.

[5] A best man is the British name for a groomsman.

[6] The tannoy is the public address system.

widowed when dad was murdered. I, (Roseanne) the youngest, was only seven at the time.

Our mum was left with nine children to raise and took on three jobs to make sure we were all provided for. She would do cleaning jobs that fit in with family life. Her family was her whole life, being a *mammy* was her whole identity.[7] Later, following the death of one of my brothers. Mum had a nervous breakdown. Due to an addiction problem, my brother had lived with her, and his death left her grief stricken and without her identity. She just didn't know how to live without being a mammy. One of her grandsons moved in with her, giving her back her role as a caregiver, and returning that precious, much needed mammy identity.

Our mum was never ill, I don't think she had seen a doctor or been in hospital, apart from when having her *weans*, until she was about 55 years old.[8] In her later years, she was diagnosed with diabetes, COPD, arthritis, and Alzheimer's Disease.[9] The Alzheimer's diagnosis came after we noticed changes in her behaviour. Our mum had always been a very laid back, quiet person and she began to become argumentative. She could be quite harsh when talking to you although there were still glimpses of her old self. She was independent and still lived at home with myself and my brother taking care of her, popping in to make sure she was ok. She always took care of her appearance despite her Alzheimer's diagnosis. First thing she always made sure was that her hair was brushed, and her false teeth were in. A sure sign of her being unwell would be the absence of her teeth.

Our mum and dad both came from large families, both had nine siblings. She had over fifty grandchildren and was the centre of our universe, she was our mammy. She was the cornerstone of our lives. She has left a massive void. Everything revolved around her.

---

[7] Mammy is a Scottish word for mum.

[8] Wean [way-n] is the west of Scotland term for a child.

[9] COPD is Chronic Obstructive Pulmonary Disease. This is an umbrella term for a group of lung conditions that cause breathing difficulties. The term includes emphysema and chronic bronchitis.

**Image 2.2** Jean Wingate.

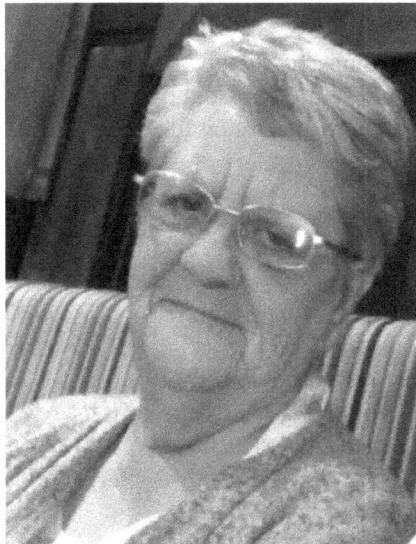

**John Francis Duffin Jackson: 8/8/1954 – 6/11/2021**

Our dad, John Jackson, was known to his friends as Johnny and was only 67 years of age when he died. He worked in a Bookmakers (bookies) writing the odds on the boards in chalk. He had five children, two daughters and three sons. I (Tracy) am the oldest. He had ten grandchildren and four great-grandchildren. He married Margaret Paul, my mum, in 1971 but they divorced three years later, something that was unusual for the time. My brother Gordon is the only one of my brothers and sisters to share my mum. We were babies when they divorced. He met Jackie in 1986 and they dated briefly before losing contact and reconnecting in 1994. They had one son together, Evan. Jackie already had two children when she met our dad: Jacqueline and Mathew. Our dad treated them like his own, he made no difference with them, and we think of them as our siblings. Dad and Jackie separated around 2003. Despite no longer being a couple, they remained great friends. Our dad was always at Jackie's for dinner, or they would go out for a meal.

Our dad was very independent and lived alone. He hated having anyone staying overnight, he liked his space, his own company. He took a pride in his appearance. He wisnae a suit man but every day he would wear a shirt with his jeans. He was very particular about how his shirts had to be ironed.

When the pandemic happened, he listened to all the advice being given, dad was the safest person ever. He had gloves in his car, he had masks in his car, he had hand sanitiser all over the house. Whenever we were going out in his car, he wore a mask and made us wear one too. He was extremely cautious with COVID, he was scared of getting it because of his health problems.[10]

We are a large close family; his family was everything to him. When he wisnae spending time with us, he could be found at the bookies, this was his second home. We had this poem written for his funeral as it said everything about who our dad was.

> *The bookie's door opens and in comes Johnny with a smile on his face and a wad of money.*
> *The sound of the puggies, and roulette wheel spinning but he's picked his horse, and he knows it's winning.[11]*
> *The only other place he'd rather be is with his kids, friends and family.*
> *A man of few words and a father like no other, a much-loved dad, granddad, great-grandad, soulmate, uncle and big brother.*
> *When we leave here today, let's all raise a toast to, Johnny in heaven with his Racing Post.[12]*
> *Family Poem (2021)*

Our dad was Johnny Jackson, a family man who liked a flutter on the horses, a man who we all miss.

**Image 2.3** John Jackson.

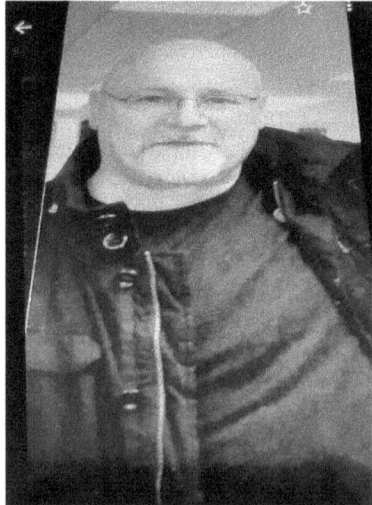

---

[10] When using the participants own words COVID-19 will be referred to as COVID.

[11] A puggie is a west of Scotland name for a slot machine.

[12] The Racing Post is a daily British betting publication. It gives the odds for horse and greyhound racing as well as betting information for other sports.

## Sam: RGN

I've been nursing for about seven or eight years now. I always wanted to be a nurse and it took a lot of hard work to get through the training, what with all the studying and placements. I was lucky when I first qualified in that I got a job in a ward I had been in as a student, and I loved it. This is not the same for everyone and I have seen newly qualified nurses being placed in wards where they feel overwhelmed. I was once moved to another ward because of staff shortages and was working alongside a young nurse who had only recently qualified. I knew her well as she had been on placement in my own ward, and I had helped to mentor her. She was incredibly stressed and said that she was just getting through each shift knowing that after three or four months she could move on. I was saddened that she was so unhappy and was counting down the days until she could leave. I could see the stress she was under, and she was almost in tears. She was underqualified for the ward they had placed her on as it had really sick patients on it that needed close monitoring, she needed mentoring and further practical training, none of which was offered to her. I was lucky, I only had to do one shift there, but she had to do many.

Even being on my own ward, can be very stressful. Staff shortages are the biggest problem. On a perfect day, we will be a team of six, four qualified staff nurses and two auxiliary nurses for around 30 patients.[13] The whole time I have been there that has never happened. On a good day, we will be working with three trained staff and two auxiliary nurses. On a bad day, we may only have two qualified nurses and one auxiliary, sometimes on night shift nurses have had to work on their own with two auxiliaries for 30 patients, this is a very unsafe practice and against everything we have to adhere to in our nursing code of conduct. I do not want to be washing patients at lunchtime, some days it could be 2 pm before we get around to them, I do not want to be telling patients I do not have the time to help them or get an auxiliary nurse to help them with walking especially when they need both our assistance. I do not want to be moved to other wards or have my colleagues moved, we are a team, and we know how each of us works, we help each other. The guilt we all feel when we call in sick, be that with a physical illness or injury or with stress. We know the pressure this will put the others under if we do not come in but some days, we are so burnt out it's the only thing we can do for our own physical and mental health.

---

[13] To ensure anonymity it was agreed with Sam that we would use 15 patients as an example. This was the staff to patient ratio when Sam worked on ward placements in another Glasgow training hospital.

We work 12-hour shifts on rotation, days, and nights. I very rarely leave the ward on time. On the day shift I should finish at 7.30 pm but some nights I do not leave until 9.30 pm. My partner gets really angry at me at times as I'm so exhausted and upset after a stressful shift, however, I'm lucky in that I live close by and have a car to get home quicker. A few times I've had to stay behind as I have to write up my notes. I cannot leave them, but I simply do not have time to do them during the day shift as I have to try prioritising patient care. On the night shift, I never take a second break, I use that time for notes or goodness knows when I would get home. I like to make sure I write everything in the notes because if I am not on shift the next day my colleagues have to be able to see exactly what has been going on with each patient.

There are times when the shift has gone well, when everyone has pulled together and we are not short staffed, those are the times I love nursing but sadly those times are becoming rarer and rarer. I don't want to leave nursing but so many of my colleagues have gone now, most of the good ones have left due to the pressures and I do not know how much longer I can continue working like this. The QEUH was heralded as a flagship modern hospital. It has all the latest equipment, but it is isolating for both staff and patients. Nurses are sent from other hospitals to help out and they talk of walking around lost and seeing no one to ask directions. Some patients, especially the elderly are alone in large rooms, they cannot even see the hustle and bustle of the ward and at times it is very difficult to get to all your patients especially if you are tied up with one or two really sick patients trying to stabilise them. Some patients have to sit in the doorways if they are at a high risk of falling, and this means we cannot treat them with dignity, which is a fundamental part of our nursing care. I look back on the wards with the four or six- bedded rooms with longing, however even then with staff shortages, I have also seen how difficult this is to manage at times.[14]

---

[14] "When I read my story before giving my permission for it to be used, I was heartbroken, it made me so sad to see how I was feeling. It had been six months since my interview. I have now left the NHS." (Sam)

Image **2.4** The QEUH.

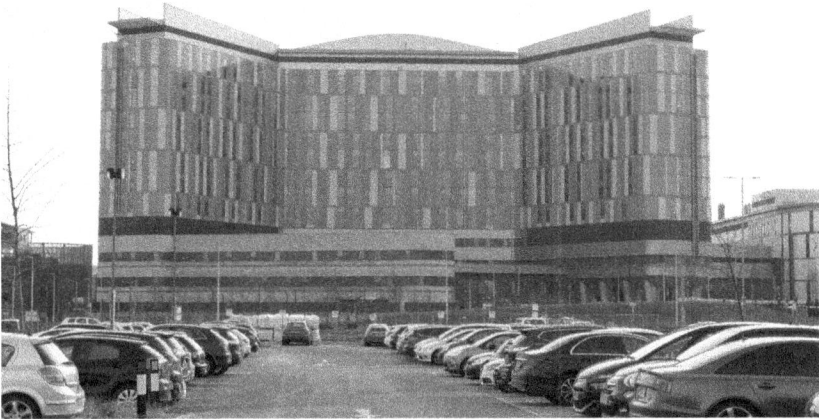

Image purchased from Shutterstock.

## Jordan: Paramedic with Scottish Ambulance Service (SAS)

For me, the most frustrating part of my job is sitting in a queue outside the hospitals with patients waiting to be admitted to A&E. This has been happening for years and years, way before COVID, queuing outside a hospital for hours and hours is not a new thing. It's important to remember that we are there because the patient needs to be seen in the hospital, quite often their GP has exhausted all other options, usually calling 999 is not the first place they go to for help. There is, however, a difference post-pandemic and that is that before we could take the patient straight into the hospital and get them checked in, we might have to queue in the corridors with them but at least we were inside with access to toilets, and it was warm. The patient would also be logged into the system. Now we have to wait outside, and of course, we have no access to toilets, in the winter it can be freezing cold and during COVID we would have to have the doors open.

The other point I want to have noted is that these patients are not logged into the system. For long enough there were no records of how long we were waiting. For that period the government were 'getting away with it 'as there were no figures to say what ambulance waiting times were. The Scottish Ambulance Service has now put in a system where we essentially clock in when we arrive at the hospital. It is not uncommon for us to be sitting outside A&E at the QEUH for five hours, it's a really good day if you are there for less than four. A long wait and then we have to return to the station to clean and re-stock the ambulance and that is another hour we are off the road. Purely from a selfish point of view, we do not get a break when we are queuing and, if there are no teams to relieve us, we have to stay well over the end of our shifts. It is only going to get worse if, or when, they close down the Inverclyde Royal Hospital (IRH). The Scottish government closed down four major Glasgow hospitals, five if you include the Southern General when they built the QEUH. The Southern used to have, I think, 18 patient bays within the A&E departments. In the QEUH they have either 20 or 22 bays, that is four extra, but they are covering four hospitals.[15] If all four of those hospitals had 18 bays, then we are 50 bays short. There have been problems with this hospital from the beginning.

We also have a drawback in the way the ambulances are allocated. It is an automated system. The dispatcher goes through a bunch of tick-box questions and an algorithm works out which patient to prioritise. The system was brought in from Canada, but we *bastardised* it to make it fit in with the NHS way of working. Calls are also colour coded, for example, a suspected heart attack is red, but someone who has had a fall is near the bottom of the list and those who are in care homes are at the very bottom. However, our response time should be 45 minutes but, as you know, it can be five hours and more. Five hours lying on the floor means that your blood starts to pool, it is not getting around your body the way it should. This system is no longer adequate, it isn't working.

Weekends get a bad name but to be honest, our worst days are Mondays, medical Mondays as they are known. A lot of unwell people will wait until Monday to see their General Practitioner (GP), but some have left it too long. Mondays are awful. For a lot of us, we are heartbroken. It is demoralising sitting and waiting outside a hospital. You cannot think about the people you should be out helping, it's too distressing. The majority of ambulance and hospital staff feel like they are just doing a job, the vocational aspect has been stripped away from us through stress and exhaustion. There is a disconnection, it is the only way to protect our mental health. We are used to seeing trauma and we learn to process that, but this is different, we can no longer do our jobs, so we have to shut off. We still know a lot of the nurses in the smaller hospitals but not at the QEUH, there is no camaraderie there and that is not healthy. There is a disconnect, if you have been waiting four hours to get a patient admitted to a bay, you start to *hate* the nurses who are *holding you up* and it is not their fault. They in turn get angry with us for berating them.

We have paramedics leaving to join the private ambulance services, these companies were unheard of ten years ago. There are so many changes, managers are no longer people who have worked their way up, they are brought

---

[15] There is a separate A&E department for children.

in, and we have managers managing managers. I have a solution, but it will not ever happen, we need to re-open some of the closed hospitals. The old Sick Children's Hospital building is still there. It is being used as a triage facility at the moment but, in my opinion, has the ability to be renovated into a teaching hospital with a fully functioning A&E department. It is soul destroying all this sitting around, I cannot let myself think about it too much, I need to look after myself.

**Dr Christina Stead**

My story is different as, firstly both my parents are still alive and, secondly, I do not have relatives who were treated in the QEUH in Glasgow. I do, however, have a family connection to the city because my maternal grandmother was born there in 1908, the daughter of a shipyard worker. She moved to England in 1911, where she married in 1934 and then raised her own family: my mother was born in 1938. Yvonne Bennett and I first met as PhD students and had often shared our experiences navigating the NHS with, and on behalf of, elderly parents. My mother spent some time in an English hospital in 2020 and, as at the QEUH, it proved difficult to navigate COVID-19 protocols and, particularly, to secure timely and effective communication with medical staff. It was interesting to note that this changed for the better when I rang and used my doctoral title. Whilst my mother recovered, and is still relatively healthy, it was a very challenging time for us as a family. She has specifically asked that her identity should be protected within the book because she still needs to access clinical services. In the interests of balance, I want to put on record that our family continues to benefit from the services provided by the NHS and that its strengths have usually far outweighed its deficiencies. A key question for me is why it is often difficult to access coordinated and properly communicated services. We will return to this point in the final chapter of the book.

When Dr Bennett mooted the idea for this book, I was keen to be a co-author, because, as illustrated by the brief details above, the experiences narrated by participants are not specific to Glasgow. Whilst certain elements are unique to the Glaswegian context, perhaps most notably the myriad issues pertaining to the physical hospital building, many others would be recognisable elsewhere in the country. As with the ongoing Covid Inquiry, it is through illuminating specific stories that we can start to build and add detail to the larger picture. This also emphasises the importance of individual lives, not least to those who have been left bereaved and mourning.

**The Importance of Storytelling**

The use of storytelling as an analytical tool is not widely used. Regardless of Maines, Pierce and Laslett informing the academic community, over fifteen years ago, that "scholars from a variety of disciplines now increasingly use it" (2008, p. 4), it remains under-utilised. I would argue that one reason behind this lack of use is that it is viewed as not being robust enough to stand up to academic scrutiny, that it is too subjective. Nevertheless, I find myself in agreement with Maines, Pierce and Laslett, that one of the delights of using storytelling is the ability to analyse a historical, socio-economic event through a personal lens:

> these analyses offer insights into human agency as seen from the inside out; as such, they can bridge the analytical gap between outside positionalities and interior worlds, between the social and the individual. (2008, p. 15).

We were aware from the beginning that using storytelling was dependent on memory and, as such, was subjective and prone to events being misremembered and/ or embellished. Any version of past events has to take into account the reasons the individual wants that rendition to be told at that moment in time. One must look at how it is being framed and what symbolic power it holds for the narrator. To combat the subjective nature of analysis we have scrutinised the participants' narrative truth alongside other sources. Maines, Pierce and Laslett proposed that although memories can alter over time that "they are shaped simultaneously by the collective, often political, narratives and individual psychological needs" (2008, p. 40). With this in mind we made the decision that using storytelling as an analytical tool was the optimum way in which our subjective data could best be explored, strengthening our constructivist approach.

By concentrating on understanding people's views of their experiences, we were able to gain a better understanding of the data we were analysing. This was especially imperative as two of our experiences took place during the COVID-19 pandemic, an unprecedented global event. Through storytelling, we were given an insight into individual experiences; allowing us to examine events from the micro to the macro. To have the ability to gain an understanding of how national decisions effected the most vulnerable within our society during a traumatic episode in their lives.

Sharing our stories is an important exercise because it allows us to connect with people who have gone through similar experiences, it is "a form of social practice" (Page, 2018, p. 206). Storytelling helps remove the isolation a negative experience can bring. Trauma and stress can affect our mental health in many ways, causing a multitude of emotional reactions, such as anxiety, depression, anger, guilt, shame, and frustration. The use of storytelling can assist in the healing process from trauma and stress. It can allow one to process and release negative emotions such as grief, guilt, and anger. But most importantly, it can bring a sense of closure. By acknowledging the traumatic experience, you can begin to disentangle, not only what has happened, but how it has affected you and how you ultimately feel about it. It can also help reframe the experience and allow one to find meaning in adversity.

Telling our stories can assist with healing, perhaps by removing the victimhood from our identities and allowing us to move forward. It helps "reinstate this powerful but isolated sequence in your life script" (Niemeyer and Stewart, 1996, p. 373). It puts these traumatic episodes into place on our life timeline, helping remove its power over feelings of guilt. Finally, it can help the storyteller connect with others who have had a similar experience, as Page noted, "[s]haring stories can bring people together" (2018, p. 1). Truth and reality can only be identified and understood through social contact; understanding that individuals are social beings and form their views and knowledge through social interaction, be that in person or through the medium of social media. The telling of our stories has enabled us to construct meaning from these traumatic experiences, it has brought us together.

My own storytelling on TikTok had many people reach out giving their accounts, and bringing a sense of community, I was not alone. Sadly, my mum was not an isolated incident of iatrogenic harm within the QEUH. The following, paraphrased, remarks are from comments and messages I received following my initial video. All shared their own tragic experiences:

- My family had a similar experience with my grandad two months ago. Following a fall, he lay on the floor with a suspected broken hip for 10 hours waiting for an ambulance. Sadly, he subsequently caught pneumonia, which we have been told was from lying on the ground. He died recently, with pneumonia being recorded as the cause of death. (R, email, 2022)

- My experience concerns my sister. She waited four and a half hours with a fractured leg. It became infected, and as a result, she had to have the leg amputated. She had to endure several more operations. During the last operation, she had a heart attack in the theatre and died. (TikTok respondent, 2022)

- My wee dad was in the QEUH and had a dreadful experience. (TikTok respondent, 2022)

- Same thing happened with a resident in the care home I work in. Seven hours for an ambulance to come. Sat outside in an ambulance for just under six hours. (TikTok respondent, 2022)

- Not only did my dad have to wait almost 40 hours in A&E last week before being seen by a doctor, but he also had a ten hour wait for a bed. (TikTok respondent, 2022)

My offloading of grief and anger had brought together a community, a community linked by tales of trauma. I felt a sense of responsibility to ensure that their voices were heard.

As time passed, I began to wonder why I chose to share such a traumatic experience with thousands of strangers, especially during a time of such vulnerability. My main reason was that I did not want to go back to my daughter's flat and offload the grief and anger, the raw emotion I was feeling. I wanted to protect Faye, to bring a sense of calm to the situation. Telling my story to strangers removed the emotional connection, these were just words, words spoken to people I would never see, never meet. There was a lack of physical distractors, I did not have to look at anyone in the eye, and I wasn't distracted by non-verbal cues. I did not have to witness their emotional response to my story. There was no attachment, it was cathartic.

On transcribing the recorded interviews, we were struck by the negative emotion that made up the majority of each narrative. The participants trusted us to present their stories to a wider audience, and for myself, Roseanne, Tracy, and Jamie-Lee, this was a way of giving our traumatic experiences a purpose. We all wanted to highlight concerns surrounding the care our elderly parents had received. All of us had come to the end of the line re formal complaints and investigations. I think that we all shared one goal in telling our stories and that was to take away the power these traumatic experiences held over feelings of guilt. My own story, as will be discussed in a subsequent chapter, allowed me to connect with people from all over the country. We will continue to use participants' own words, share our stories, and use our voices in the following two chapters. Basia Cummings once said, "memory is always slippery, in grief even more so" (2023, podcast). I would argue that in the grief I experienced following the trauma, my memory remained solid. However, I must consider that I recorded the events in a series of three-minute videos, so I can refresh my memory at any time.

As mentioned, my storytelling took place over the social media platform TikTok. This proved to have effects that I did not foresee. Social media is not a straightforward medium (McMahon, 2019; Page, 2018). Once you have shared your narrative you have limited control over who views, comments, or likes your content. As McMahon points out, "while social media is personal, like a diary or a self-help book, it is essentially a public transmission." (2019, p. 93). The audience that can view your content and listen to your story is not random but "driven by algorithms" (Page, 2018, p. 119). This ensures your content is viewed by people with similar cultural identities, interests, ages, and social demographics. My initial video had over 300,600 views with 2,607 comments. This was something I had not considered, and although the majority of the comments were sympathetic, some were not, adding to the trauma.

# Chapter Three

# NHS Scotland in Critical Care

Yvonne Bennett

The idea that people's lives and experiences contribute to our understanding of society is not new, use of life story data has a relatively long tradition within ethnography. We have utilised this method to analyse the experiences of both the patients' families and the healthcare workers. Lutova et al. remind us that:

> [d]ue to its extremely personal and sensitive nature, health care has its own unique, context-specific characteristics. These characteristics make health care an interesting field for examining experiences (2019, p. 1).

During such an emotional period in some people's lives, it was important to seize the complexities of lived experiences while respecting personal space and boundaries. Personal stories exist in the social and historical backgrounds from which they emerged and sit alongside public narratives. As this book is examining a specific time within history, during and just following a global pandemic our analysis has used both personal narratives and other sources such as professional and governmental documentation. This chapter will analyse the data from the two staff participants, discussing the identified themes: staff shortages, stress, trauma, and disillusionment. One aim of this chapter is to attempt to answer the question posed by McLardy-Smith in 2022 "[t]he NHS as an employer; is it worth saving?" (p. 31). As constructivist theory can be used to inform policies, practices, and interventions related to topics such as healthcare, it further strengthened our decision to use a constructivist approach.

Scotland has a rich history in the field of medicine, with the first UK medical school established in Edinburgh in 1726, followed by Glasgow in 1744. In 1809, William Ferguson was the first known black student to attend Edinburgh University School of Medicine. Half a century later, Africanus Horton, the son of freed slaves, also graduated from this prestigious school. In 1928, the Scottish Scientist, Alexander Fleming discovered penicillin at St Mary's Hospital in London. This accidental discovery changed the world of medicine as it treated what were then potentially fatal infections. In 1948 the NHS was born, brought to fruition by Aneurin Bevan. He wrote, "no society can legitimately call itself civilised if a sick person is denied medical aid because of a lack of means." (Bevan, cited in McLardy-Smith, 2022, p. 20). The NHS patient charter expounds that every individual who comes into contact with it should always be treated with respect and dignity, regardless of whether they are a patient, carer, or member of staff.[1] With this in mind, the NHS seeks to ensure that all of its organisations, when delivering services, value and respect the different needs of individuals without any bias. The NHS is founded on a common set of principles and values that bind together the people it serves, the patients, their friends and families and the staff who work for it. (Department of Health 2015). The key to providing such care is good communication as this connects with the respect and dignity that individual patients and their families must be treated with. The business of the NHS goes beyond simply providing clinical care and includes making people feel valued and that their concerns are important; "[t]he NHS belongs to the people" (Department of Health 2015).

Sadly, in the 75 years since its inception, the NHS has failed to live up to all that it promised. Coleman argues that the cause of its decline: excess waiting lists, staff shortages and sub-standard hospital buildings, is due to an increase in bureaucratical authority "while at the same time diminishing the position of patients" (2022, p. 4). One cannot argue that running the enormous institution that is the NHS requires people with managerial and financial expertise. NHS Greater Glasgow and Clyde Health Board (NHSGGC) has an annual budget of £3.3 billion. It is the largest health board in Scotland, serving a population of around 1.3 million people, and employing over 43,500 staff in 35 hospitals, GP surgeries, health centres, dental practices and clinics. In addition to business leaders, NHS Scotland also needs people with experience in clinical departments and wards, people who have worked at the *coal face*. At the heart of the NHS Scotland are the patients and those who treat and care for them, "if a civilised society is one that protects the weak, then it must have a satisfactory health care delivery service" (McLardy-Smith, 2022, p. 29). However, it seems that in twenty-first century Scotland, the vulnerable population, particularly the elderly, are not receiving the service they need, and those who look after them are growing more disheartened.

## Malaise within NHS Scotland

The NHS does extremely well in the management of acute trauma. My husband John has often said, "the NHS is amazing at saving lives, it's afterwards that they let you down", a saying that comes from personal experience.[2] However,

---

[1] The NHS patient charter for England is reviewed every ten years. The devolved assemblies of the UK have set their own NHS patient charters which follow a similar vein and are also regularly reviewed.

[2] Our eldest son was critically ill when he was 15 years old due to a rare complication to a virus. He has since made a good recovery.

McLardy-Smith argues that even in times of medical emergencies, the provision of care is not equal. He points out, when discussing A&E's excellent treatment of fractures, that:

> there are exceptions which again involve the people whose life is not obviously going to be immediately changed by the fracture. These are people whose quality of life is already dramatically diminished by some co-morbidity, the most common of which is senility... hip fractures in the elderly are a common and quite frequently terminal event. Although outcomes have improved somewhat, it remains the case that they are often fixed or treated by some form of hip replacement on an 'out of hours' operating list for emergencies and performed by relatively junior trainees. (2022, p. 25).

Relatively junior trainees would be in theatre with the lead surgeon, elderly individuals would be placed at the end of an operating schedule and using them for teaching purposes seems callous. This represents an inadequate healthcare delivery, and it serves as a clear example of iatrogenic disease.

Peter McLardy-Smith is himself a consultant surgeon with many years of experience working in the NHS and discusses in his 2022 book *Eden is Burning* not only regional variations to care but also variations between local hospitals, adding that if he required surgery, he has the inside knowledge to know who he would have carry out the operation and more importantly who he would not. He further noted that "for better, or worse, that type of *inside* information is not widely available to the general public" (2022, p. 26).

NHS managers are facing pressure when their performance is judged based on meeting specific targets. However, many of these managers lack *hands-on* experience in clinical settings. How can people manage medical clinicians when they have limited knowledge of how and what each clinician does? Historically, managers had worked through the ranks. The old ward matron had begun his/her career as a student nurse. The manager of a rehabilitation ward had trained and worked as a physiotherapist, occupational therapist, or speech therapist. Over the past few decades, this has no longer been the case with people being employed for their managerial skills and expertise. There is a preconception that NHS Scotland is now becoming top-heavy with those in managerial positions:

> managers are no longer people who have worked their way up, they are brought in, and we have managers managing managers. (Jordan, 2022).

Previously, those in leadership positions had a clear understanding of the clinical area they oversaw from a professional perspective. They possessed clinical knowledge that allowed them to recognise that shifting a nurse from a general surgical unit to a high-dependency A&E receiving unit would be an extremely stressful change, similar to expecting a physiotherapist to substitute for an occupational therapist. Yet management today appears to "think of nurses as being an amorphous inter-changeable mass." (McLardy-Smith, 2022, p. 51). A main theme that ran through Sam's narrative was that of being moved to other wards to cover staff shortages. This was especially stressful if it was a ward that they had no prior experience with or one in which they felt undertrained. Sam spoke of their concerns about being moved:

> I was getting put in unsafe situations. I got sent to a cardiology ward. OK, I'm a medical nurse but I don't work in cardiology.... I don't really know a lot about it.... there were people on sliding scales and patients on monitors and I was like 'well I can't make head nor tail of them so I'm not doing them at all'.... I just felt like I was getting put into unsafe situations all the time. I actually had to take time out. I went off work for two weeks sick, just the stress.... I cannot do this anymore. (Sam, 2023).

It can be considered that in this situation, Sam suffered an iatrogenic injury due to managerial negligence. There was also potential harm to the patients as Sam lacked the knowledge to care for their complex needs.

Sam also reported that some nurses are moved to the QEUH from other hospitals. This is problematic as the QEUH is NHSGGC's acute receiving hospital and Scotland's major trauma hospital. As a result, the QEUH has critically ill patients sent to it from, not only other hospitals within the district, but from other health board areas. The nearest hospital to the QEUH is Gartnavel General Hospital (the hospital I trained in), and Sam confirmed that this is where nurses are moved from. Although this is a large teaching hospital it does not have an A&E department, therefore admissions are scheduled and patients, although sick, tend to be more stable. The wards also have a significant number of elderly patients in need of rehabilitation or waiting to be discharged, with a considerable portion falling under the category referred to as *bed blockers*. The question posed at this juncture is why managers would transfer nurses from another hospital, were there no available staff within the QEUH that could be moved? A problem with nurses coming from Gartnavel was that it could take an hour for them to arrive on the ward, an hour of nursing time lost, and patients being cared for in an unsafe environment, vulnerable to iatrogenic disease due to dangerous staffing ratios.

Being moved to another ward is not a new occurrence and was something I experienced when working in the 1980s. However, it was not a regular event, and I was only moved to another ward when I was a student nurse, and they needed an extra pair of hands to carry out basic tasks. I was never moved to a ward if I was underqualified to work there. I was also never moved when I was a Registered General Nurse (RGN), I remained in the post I was employed for. This no longer happens:

> [w]ard nurses have applied for a post on a specific unit: they would always be prepared to cover another ward in difficult circumstances, but they do not want to find themselves shunted off, with no prior notice to a different ward every time they come into work. (McLardy-Smith, 2022, p. 51).

Moving staff in such a manner helps hide chronic staff shortages, but could there be another motive behind such staffing tactics? McLardy-Smith offers that "everyone is left feeling lonely and vulnerable, disempowered with no sense of team identity. A classic ploy for keeping a workforce under control." (2022, p. 51). One consequence of moving staff is that it leads to further staff shortages, as people who feel unhappy being moved from ward to ward with no warning simply leave, something Sam reluctantly did. It has been reported by the interim director for the Royal College of Nursing (RCN) that the staffing levels have become so low that nurses cannot take a break. They further added that "almost 9 in 10 nursing staff said that staffing levels on their last shift, when surveyed, were not sufficient to meet the needs of patients" (Macgill and Pringle, 2023). Could it be that the stress of never knowing when or where you will be moved to has a part to play in the increased suicide rates among nurses and other health workers? (Mars et al., 2020; Riley and Causer, 2023)

Riley and Causer noted that "[t]he suicide rate for health workers is 24% higher than in the general population. This is largely explained by increased levels of suicide among female nurses, female doctors, and male paramedics" (2023, p. 36). Further research in this field is essential: studies are necessary to find out why female nurses and doctors are more likely to commit suicide than their peers. This high statistic for women medics is concerning, especially when one considers that three-quarters of all suicides are committed by men, with it, sadly, being the main cause of death in men under 50 years of age (Sutherland, 2018). A large nationwide study is required to gain an understanding of the causes behind such a striking statistic. Suicide within the ambulance service will be examined later in this chapter, but one cause appears to be low morale within the workplace. Whatever the reasons behind such high rates of suicide, one must recognise that "[e]very death by suicide impacts approximately 80 – 135 people…. 1 in 30 of whom may be deeply impacted and so can be considered bereaved" (Riley and Causer, 2023, p. 36). A death by suicide affects family, friends, and colleagues, however, within the workplace, many NHS staff felt they were expected to carry on, with no time allocated to either attend the funeral or to have time off to grieve (Riley and Causer, 2023).

Moving staff to wards that they have little or no experience in can have serious consequences when it comes to drug administration. As we were beginning the research for this book, the Scottish media was reporting the death of a patient through a misadministration of drugs. Martin Weldon, 36 years of age, was a patient in ICU in the QEUH. Mr. Weldon was diabetic and had suffered a catastrophic brain injury following a hypoglycaemic episode. It was widely reported, by the Scottish media, that, despite having a long rehabilitation period ahead of him, he was showing signs of recovery. At the time, the Scottish media was reporting the death as *sudden and unexplained* but also stated that he had been given a lethal dose of another patient's medication. His death underwent a police investigation.[3] Although an inquiry has still to report its findings over the death of Mr. Weldon, whilst carrying out the interviews for this investigation, all the participants related the story. Sam mentioned that in the incident, a nurse, who had been relocated to the ICU from another ward, administered the drug by mistake; however, this information has not been officially verified. Research carried out by Carvalho dos Santos and Ceolim in Brazil is pertinent to this study of NHS Scotland. They wrote that:

> [t]here are several types of iatrogeny committed by the nursing team, and the most common are related to medications: omission of doses, administration in incorrect concentration, application at inappropriate times, and through inappropriate route, medication administration to the wrong patient as well as application of incorrect drugs due to inappropriate substitutions or doubts regarding the transcription. (2007, p. 809).

As will be discussed in the following chapter, my mum also had a problem with drug administration. She had her operation cancelled after being given her anti-coagulant in error the night before. The nurse who was on duty was from another ward and did not know that the drug should be withheld prior to surgery. The doctor on call was only days into her first post as a junior doctor, and did not know to cancel the drug on the drug chart. When I complained about my mum's treatment in the QEUH, I was left with the impression that the doctor was reprimanded over the incident despite my reporting that this was down to dangerous nurse management practice. For that reason, I regret my complaint. When I was researching the death of Mr. Weldon, I found a newspaper article about my mum, one I hadn't known was published. Being given the wrong medication in error is not the only cause of iatrogenic harm for the elderly, Zazzara et al. (2020) noted that the complex medical needs of the elderly can lead to adverse drug reactions, especially for those who are

---

[3] On May 30th 2024 the nurse responsible for administering the wrong medication to Mr Weldon was charged with culpable homicide.

categorised as frail. This, it must be noted, is a global problem. Zazzara et al.'s research concluded that the complex medical needs underline "the necessity of a holistic approach" (2020, p. 47) when prescribing multiple medications to this cohort.

Ward and Brady (2022) wrote a newspaper article highlighting just how dangerous the situation was at the QEUH due to staff shortages. Patients' lives were being put in danger, and between 18th July – 18th August 2022, two patients lost their lives. Information obtained through a FOI request noted that a total of 336 incidents that resulted in patient harm were "blamed on either staffing levels or an inappropriate skill mix'" (Ward and Brady, 2022).[4] These incidents were deemed to have been avoidable. All of such incidents are recorded on NHS Scotland's Datix system, and all of the aforementioned incidents were recorded as "staffing/inappropriate skill mix issues" (Ward and Brady, 2022). Sam spoke of the importance of using the Datix system to record any changes to a patient that could be seen as iatrogenic, such as the development of a pressure sore:

> I actually think they are sick of me because I Datix everything. Some of the lassies don't bother but…. It's a lot of work; it is extra time you need to take out to do it, but they need to know this is happening. So, I Datix and record everything. I will put "patient care not done due to staff shortages". This is just what I record, every single time, because I'm not going to take the brunt of it. (Sam, 2023).

Sam was also of the opinion that since they started using the Datix system to record every incident that was caused by low staffing levels management was moving staff from their ward on fewer occasions.

Unsafe staffing numbers are not restricted to the QEUH. This is a problem that affects the UK as a whole. In March 2022, The Royal College of Nursing carried out a survey of its members into staffing levels.[5] The subsequent report: *Nursing under unsustainable Pressures (UK)*, was published in June of that year, with separate publications released which examined the data from the individual nations. The following findings are from the Scottish publication and responses from registered nurses working in NHS Scotland:

- 86% said there were insufficient numbers of staff per shift to meet the needs and dependencies of the patients.

- 70% reported that patient safety was compromised. In the UK as a whole, this number was 62%.

---

[4] I requested data relating to the number of iatrogenic incidents recorded in other HNS Scotland Trusts during the same period. This was a FOI request that I received no reply to.

[5] This is the most recent survey into staffing levels.

- 62% felt exhausted following a shift, this is higher than the UK number at 54%.

- 62% were unable to take breaks during 12-hour shifts.

- 62% continued working after the end of a shift so that work could be completed.

- 16% felt that their ward was sufficiently staffed to allow the appropriate level of care to be given to patients.

- 69% felt they were able to raise concerns over staffing numbers, however, only 35% of these were acted on.

- At the time of the report there were 6700 nursing and midwifery vacancies within NHS Scotland. (The Royal College of Nursing, 2022).

The RCN has stated that the number of student nurses must be increased to help with staffing issues in the long term. This is paramount as around 34% of nurses and midwives are aged 51+years and, as a consequence, in the next decade, a large proportion of nurses will retire. Younger nurses are a necessity to fill future staffing voids (NMC, 2023).

The shortage of nursing was a topic that came up in the comments of my TikTok videos:

- An NHS worker told me that they saw the shortages firsthand. They added that they never thought they would see it in such a state. With people leaving in droves due to a lack of decent wages and support (TikTok respondent, 2022)

- Another TikTok user informed me that the Langlands unit (geriatric unit) in QEUH only had one trained nurse per ward on Sunday. (TikTok respondent, 2022)

There had been, since the pandemic, a three-fold increase in people interested in a nursing career, however, in the last year, numbers are dropping again, with "a fall of 16%" in Scottish university applications in 2023 (RCN, 2023). Nonetheless, staff recruitment is only the first stepping stone to overcoming chronic staff shortages, recruitment must be matched by retention, and this is especially true of student nurses. I submitted an FOI to the Higher Education Statistics Agency (HESA) requesting data on the numbers of students who:

1. are accepted onto a nurse training programme
2. numbers who complete said programme
3. numbers who continue to work for NHS Scotland.

Scotland has free university education for Scottish students, but due to costs incurred by the universities, the number of places is capped, with 1200 places to be removed for the academic year 2024/25. The majority of students taking up places at Scottish universities are fee paying, either from the other UK nations or worldwide. When the UK was a part of the European Union (EU), the free places had to be shared with other EU students as part of an EU directive. I was interested to discover if, when qualified, students returned to their home countries. Unfortunately, HESA could not supply me with this data and to be furnished with a custom set of data was extremely expensive. What I was able to ascertain that 84% of students who studied dentistry or medicine enter the NHS. When it came to students who studied for other health/medical degrees, such as nursing or physiotherapy, the number was lower at 78%. (HESA, 2023).[6] These numbers may take into account students from countries outside the UK returning home.

Recent data shows that when it comes to nursing degrees, "two thirds of students in Scotland have considered dropping out of their courses" (Church, 2023). Interestingly the number one reason given is financial problems, with around 99% stating that money causes them concern (Church, 2023; Jackson, 2023; RCN, 2023). The RCN report Nursing Student Finance tells us that:

> [n]ursing students across Scotland are facing serious financial pressures that are having a significant impact on their education, financial security and physical and mental wellbeing…providing nursing students across the UK with appropriate financial support is key to attracting the next generation into nursing and addressing the nursing workforce crisis" (2023, p. 5).

Many student nurses supplement their nursing bursary by taking on paid work within the NHS bank system or private nursing agencies.[7] However, this is not a satisfactory solution as, due to the hours required for study and being on placement, opportunities to take on paid work are limited. The RCN has implored the Scottish Government to increase the monies given to the bursary programme.

Sam was saddened when moved to another ward to find a newly qualified nurse working there who was crossing off the days until they could leave and

---

[6] This was the most recent data available and encompassed the academic years 2019/2020; 2021/2022. See https://www.hesa.ac.uk/data-and-analysis/sb266/figure-1

[7] Nursing students receive a bursary of £1000 for their first three years of training. For those who take on a fourth year the bursary drops to £7500 for that final year. There are also other grants available. See: https://www.gov.scot/publications/support-paramedic-nursing-midwifery-students-scotland-2022-23/pages/4/

find a job elsewhere. A nurse who had only been qualified for approximately a month was already disillusioned. The loss of younger, less experienced staff was highlighted by the Nursing and Midwifery Council in their 2023 report *Leavers' Survey 2022*. They noted that out of those leaving 19% had been on the register for less than 10 years. Further examination of the data revealed that within the 18-34 year age group only 26% were not considering leaving the profession (NMC, 2023). The top reasons given for considering leaving were:

**Figure 3.1** Reasons for Leaving the Nursing Profession in 18–34 age group.

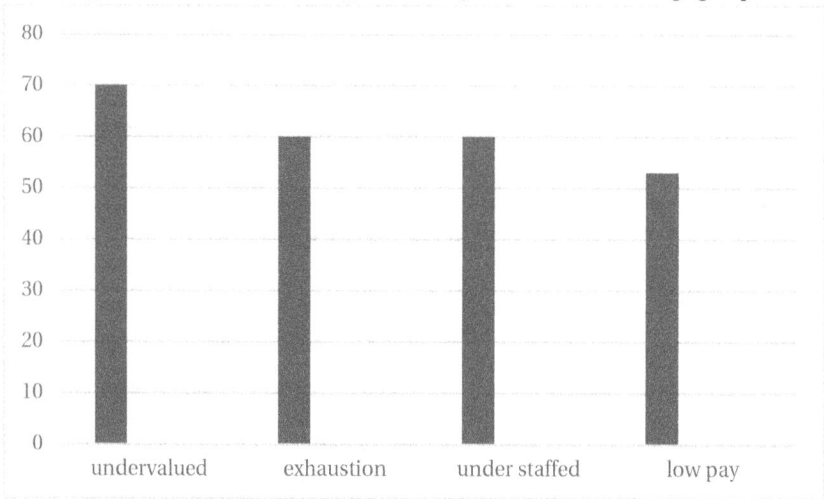

Data from: Nursing and Midwifery Council (2023) Leavers' survey 2022. Available at: https://www.nmc.org.uk/news/news-and-updates/record-number-of-nurses-midwives-and-nursing-associates/. Accessed: 10th April 2024.

Despite it not being the number one reason for leaving, could an increase in wages help keep staff? I would argue that, although a wage that reflects both your skill set and the work you do, is paramount. Without rock-solid support from management, staff will continue to abandon the NHS. The NMC notes that wages have not kept up with inflation. NHS Scotland has increased nurse wages by an average of 6.5%, however, Scotland has the highest income tax of the UK nations so, in relative terms, the increase is offset by taxation, especially for those in the higher bands. I became aware, from conversations the morning of my mum's accident, that nurses were leaving their jobs within the hospital and returning the following week as agency staff. This led to a problem of agency staff feeling ostracised. Nurses doing the same job for much more money led to feelings of resentment, with Sam reporting that some agency staff were treated horribly by the other nurses on the ward. Unfortunately, due to budget cuts, some Scottish Health Boards are requesting that staff recruitment be slowed down as there are insufficient funds in their budgets to support an increase in staffing levels (Macgill and Pringle, 2023). NHS England has set out a retention strategy which looks to help nurses to work for longer, creating career pathways as well as allowing for flexible working patterns (NHS England, 2020). NHS Scotland does not have such a strategy in place despite repeated appeals by the RCN (Devereux, 2023).

### Low Morale

A low morale theme ran through all narratives, whether from hospital staff at the time of my mum's accident, comments left on TikTok, or through semi-structured interviews later on:

> Morale at the QEUH is so low. I have friends who work there, and they complain that they are overworked. The numbers of staff who have been signed off work due to sickness is shocking. (TikTok respondent, 2022).

This staff crisis is also noted by McLardy-Smith "[w]ithin the NHS the biggest problem, in my opinion, is collapsing morale. It is tiring and very depressing to be constantly fighting a losing battle against a firewall." (2022, p. 29). As previously mentioned, anonymity was of utmost importance when talking to the two staff members who agreed to take part in this research project; initially, six members of staff had expressed an interest, but four dropped out due to concerns about their jobs. It was paramount that neither participant could be identified from their stories, as a result, we used gender-neutral pseudonyms and they/them pronouns. Both participants told us that being a whistle-blower was a sackable offence. This fear of speaking out correlated with Coleman's findings when he wrote "[a]nyone who questions the establishment must be ignored and, if they persist, they must be crushed, suppressed, vilified and ostracised." (2022, p. 17). Yet freedom of speech must be protected within NHS Scotland, it is through staff highlighting issues that those receiving care are protected; one way in which iatrogenic harm can be prevented. I approached the Members of the Scottish Parliament's (MSP) health spokesman for all six political parties with questions relating to whistleblowing[8] I sent the following email:

> I am an independent sociology researcher, and I am, at present, writing a book on NHS Scotland with a particular focus on the Queen Elizabeth University Hospital. I am doing so after a traumatic experience at the

---

[8] The Scottish Parliament Building is situated in the Holyrood district of Edinburgh and is commonly known as Holyrood. The Scottish Parliament is the devolved legislature taking responsibility for devolved issues such as law, health, taxation and education. It comprises of 129 democratically elected members. The six parties are Scottish Labour, Scottish Conservative and Unionist Party, Scottish Liberal Democrats, Scottish National Party (SNP), and the Scottish Green Party.

hospital with my mum in August 2022. After going public with this experience, I was approached by others with similar stories to tell. As a result, I am writing a book highlighting the unequal approach to health care for our elderly. I was approached by numerous members of NHS Scotland staff but all, bar two, were reluctant to be interviewed due to concerns about whistleblowing. Can I ask if you are aware of staff concerns regarding the unequal treatment of the elderly within NHS Scotland? Are you aware of a culture of fear amongst staff regarding speaking out? Is it an un/written rule that to speak out results in instant dismissal? Would you be happy for your replies to be used within the book? This book is academic and is being published by Vernon Press.

Dr Yvonne Bennett.

I had spoken on three occasions to the head of the Scottish Labour Party, Anas Sarwar, about my mum, her treatment, and this book. Although sympathetic, his busy schedule meant he was unable to contribute to this research and suggested I reach out to the health spokesman. As I do not live in Scotland, I was unsure if any of those I contacted would reply. There were varying times for their responses. The first response took only three days and came from Dr Sandesh Gulhanne, the health spokesman for the Scottish Conservative and Unionist Party. He kindly offered to do a 30-minute telephone conversation. We had an interesting conversation, but he requested that everything remain *off the record*, he is still employed, as a GP, within NHS Scotland. Although I cannot print our conversation, he did confirm many of the things other staff members had reported. None of the other MSPs replied to my email, although MSP, Cabinet Secretary for NHS Recovery, Health, and Social Care, forwarded on my email to the Directorate for Health Workforce. She attached NHS Scotland's protocol for whistleblowing as a reply, see appendix 2.

NHS staff being dissuaded about raising concerns about un-safe practices is not a new issue. Sirrs notes that for decades:

> [d]octors speaking up about errors, avoidable deaths and other failures in hospitals could face severe repercussions. There have been many high-profile cases of whistleblowing doctors being victimised, dismissed from their jobs or even facing spurious referral to the GMC [General Medical Council] after raising concerns. (2023, p. 11).[9]

Whistleblowers are protected under Scottish employment law. NHS Scotland has a set of whistleblowing standards which states "all NHS service providers to

---

[9] The GMC is a regulatory body that holds records for all doctors registered in the UK. It sets standards for practice as well as investigating complaints against doctors. It has the power to strike a doctor from the medical register.

handle concerns that are raised with them, and which meet the definition of a 'whistleblowing concern'" (NHS Scotland, 2021). If, following a complaint, the whistleblower remains unsatisfied then they can escalate the complaint to the Independent National Whistleblowing Officer. Nonetheless, all NHS Scotland staff, who contacted me, voiced concerns over whistleblowing. Whilst acknowledging that they were protected under employment laws they were of the opinion that to raise concerns would see their career prospects falter. They also mentioned that to speak to an outside organisation, for example, the media, or to post or comment on concerns on social media was a sackable offense. Regarded as bringing NHS Scotland into disrepute. A majority of the staff spoke of a culture of bullying from and fear of QEUH management.[10]

Bullying within the nursing community is not restricted to NHS Scotland but is an international problem, with Bambi et al. reporting that "87.4% of nurses worldwide across 24 countries were victims of bullying" (2018, p. 51). Nurses reported that the main perpetrators of bullying were their supervisors, although such behaviour could also come from colleagues as well as patients and their families (Shorey and Wong 2021). Bullying can take many forms and can be difficult to identify. Behaviours range from exclusion and abuse to limited career progression. The effects felt by those being bullied vary from the physical to the mental, with as Bambi et al. noting "absenteeism 1.5 times higher in comparison to non-victim peers" (2018, p. 51). Sadly, the majority of those who reported being bullied were in relatively new positions, and as such, research has shown that these are the nurses most likely to leave the profession (Bambi et al., 2018; Shorey and Wong, 2021). These findings are supported by Jackson, who carried out research into the reasons why midwifery students left the programme before qualification. Jackson put forward that students spoke of intimidation from both lectures and mentors, which "indicted a dysfunctional culture where some midwives display bullying characteristics" (2023, p. 217). She noted a culture of silence surrounding bullying, with students using silence as a survival mechanism.

During my research into the bacterial infections which caused the deaths of children (see Chapter Five) I came across a newspaper article which was initiated by a whistleblower. The article looked at how a senior manager at the QEUH spoke of a father whose daughter was receiving cancer treatment at the hospital. The teenager had acquired a life-threatening infection, which was believed to have been caused by the hospital environment. The senior manager spoke of the father in a disparaging way to staff members. The whistleblower made several complaints to the QEUH's chief executive about the manager, but none were upheld. They subsequently left the NHS and were quoted in the

---

[10] To maintain the anonymity of one of our staff participants we cannot discuss any incidents they mentioned during their interview as this would make them identifiable.

newspaper as saying "the irony is working for the NHS made me ill. That wasn't the job itself, it was the toxic culture." (Aitkin, 2023). A statement from the NHSGGC said:

> [w]e take our responsibility to our staff very seriously and we are dedicated to supporting them to raise issues and concerns should they need to". It added: "We can confirm that when these allegations were raised initially, robust HR protocols were followed and a full investigation was undertaken, however, it would be inappropriate to comment further about individual cases. (Aitkin, 2023).

The 2000 AOWAM report noted the need to remove "the wall of silence" (Sirrs, 2023, p. 3) when it came to making complaints about the treatment and care received in the NHS. The complaints system needed to be simplified, and this included complaints coming from medical practitioners re practices they saw as being contributory to patient harm. Yet, change seems to be slow in the making. In Scotland the organisation Healthcare Improvement Scotland (HIS) is a designated organisation where people can make formal complaints. It aims to guide people through the complaint procedure, simplifying the process. They assess if they can deal with the complaint and if not, they furnish the complainant with the information needed to take the complaint forward. If the complaint can be handled by HIS then they will carry out an initial assessment and will liaise with the relevant NHS Scotland board. One important point they make is that:

> [t]he assessment process is designed to be independent. We do not act on behalf of the individual who has raised the concerns. We do not look at individual patient care or incidents. We consider the concerns raised within the context of the systems/processes within which they sit. We also consider the potential impact on patient safety/quality of care in the delivery of that service. (HIS, 2024).

HIS has come under criticism when, in March 2024, the Scottish media reported that, in May 2023, 29 emergency medicine consultants had written an open letter to HIS noting serious concerns over patient safety due to un-safe staffing levels. They offered to provide 18 months' worth of evidence, but, not only did HIS refuse their offer, but they did also not engage with the consultants. In August of 2023, HIS wrote to the NHSGGC chief executive, informing her that they were closing the investigation as "it was satisfied there was awareness and oversight of the issues and of the performance of the emergency department'." (McArdle, 2024). They came to this conclusion after management at the hospital simply said they were aware of the concerns. The consultants have since been offered an apology.

Nurses complaining of feeling burnt out by working conditions are not restricted to the UK and the NHS. Kelly et al. wrote that, in the United States, "[a]s many as half of the nursing workforce are experiencing burnout with the likelihood of personal consequence, job dysfunction, and potential risk to patients." (2021, p. 96) an indicator of iatrogenic disease. The three symptoms of burnout noted by Kelly et al. are described by nurses such as Sam. These are exhaustion, cynicism and a reduction in personal achievement:

> Sometimes I've got back here (home) exhausted at ten o'clock at night...I'm meant to finish at half past seven (7.30 pm) …. And I went and got her (charge nurse on a ward they had been moved to) and I said, 'I don't know this patient and she was like 'well that is just what he's in with all the time' and she went back to her break (patient was having seizures) …. And you feel bad, you feel so bad because you can't deal with it. (Sam, 2023).

I also received similar comments on TikTok, with staff informing me that:

- As nurses we can't care for patients the way we want to and the way they deserve. This is so upsetting and demoralising. (TikTok respondent, 2022)

- Drs and nurses are trying their best, and the majority of us still care. However, we are short staffed and there's only so much we can do. (TikTok respondent, 2022)

At the time of their interview, Sam had applied for a non-nursing job within NHSGGC. They explained that the constant stress over long working hours, being short-staffed, concerns over being moved and being unable to provide the level of care they felt was appropriate was proving detrimental to their physical and mental health. This correlates with the findings of Kelly et al. "[n]urses may feel reduced personal accomplishment and a lack of job satisfaction in response to job-related stressors and eventually leave their position" (2021, p. 97). Six months after their interview, Sam left the NHS, their way of combating the iatrogenic disease that had affected them over the past year. Not only had their mental health declined, but they were also suffering from a back injury, caused by moving patients alone whilst attending to their personal hygiene needs. Moving a patient on one's own, should not happen, and, throughout training, nurses are instructed that such procedures require two people. The blame lies at your door if you do otherwise and damage your back. Unfortunately, with staff shortages, and time at a premium, nurses do take the risk. Sam's line manager had been extremely good when they were ill, referring them to Occupational Health for their back issue and their declining mental health.

Stress is a major cause of sick days within NHS Scotland. The Scottish government has set a target of achieving a sickness absence rate of 4%. Their latest published data shows a rate that is running at 5.69% for 2022.[11] The rate varies from health board to health board, with NHS Shetland having the lowest rate at 4.29%, NHSGGC coming in at 6.28%, third highest after NHS Lanarkshire at 6.61% and NHS 24 at 8.48%. NHS Scotland's rates are higher than those in England, where the rate for March 2023 was 4.9%, dropping by 1.1% in 12 months. Again, there were variations between health authorities with the Northwest Region having the highest rate at 5.7%, still considerably lower than Scotland. NHS England reported, "[a]nxiety/stress/depression/other psychiatric illness was the most reported reason for sickness, accounting for over 507,100 full-time equivalent days lost and 24.2% of all sickness absence in March 2023." (NHS Digital, 2023). Stress was a factor in the sudden illness of a colleague of Sam's, stress brought on by being moved to another ward with no notice:

> One of the other staff nurses (RGN) went over to one of the other wards and she felt ill. She ended up in A&E. They thought perhaps she was having a stroke…. So, they gave her aspirin, and they were treating her in A&E and all that. Anyway, it turned out it was stress. (Sam, 2023).

A lack of staff seems to be at the centre of many of the day to day running problems encountered in NHS Scotland. As was noted by Tracy and her daughter Jamie-Lee, the organisation outsources amenities to the private sector.[12] This can be any service from operations to diagnostic testing or rehabilitation. Nonetheless, it is important to emphasise that no private company will assume responsibilities within NHS Scotland without a profit motive. This utilisation is, in my opinion, extremely short-sighted. While it may decrease patient waiting times, it will do so at a financial expense that diminishes NHS Scotland's cash flow. Anderson noted that, during the initial stages of the pandemic, payment to the private sector saw "[a] total of £30.6m has been paid up to March 2021, according to figures released in response to freedom of information requests, while a contract notice posted online suggests the overall amount may approach £40m." (October 2023). Initially, this had been a short-term solution to the long waiting lists that had occurred during the initial wave of the pandemic. I placed a Freedom of Information Request (FOI) to the Scottish Government regarding the total cost of using private hospitals for the year January 2022 – January 2023. I received the standard reply that the information I was after was not available. This had been

---

[11] This data was last updated on 8th September 2022 and does not include COVID-19 related absences as these are reported using a different system. Data available from https://www.gov.scot/publications/nhsscotland-performance-against-ldp-standards/pages/sickness-absence/.

[12] I am using NHS Scotland, but I must point out that all of the home nations outsource to private hospitals this is not a practice that only the NHS Scotland undertakes.

one of answers I received when making FOI requests, the other was that it wasn't in the public's interest to release the information.

At the time of their interview, Sam had joined a private agency to do extra shifts alongside their job in the QEUH. They wanted to try agency work before fully committing. They explained this was something a lot of their colleagues did. It had both positives and negatives as, although the pay was better, and nurses could pick their hours, they lost out on holiday and sick pay as well as pension contributions. Jordan also spoke of the number of private ambulance services that were now available, something I had used for both of my parents:

> [y]ou see more and more.... They are brilliant and if it wasn't for them our situation would be a lot worse, they do a lot of transfers. Not even 10 years ago you never saw a private ambulance.... Almost every day you're thinking that's a new sign (insignia) and there's obviously business because we can't cope because we are sitting outside hospitals for too long. (Jordan, 2022).

When carrying out research for this book I came across Remedy Insourcing, a private agency that advertised their services to the NHS. This company, as do many others, offer a solution to long waiting lists, but at a cost. These companies also employ staff who have left the NHS, engaging staff who are fully trained, Sam and Jordan both spoke of colleagues moving to the private sector for better work and wage conditions. When sitting beside my mum as she slept, I put on my sociologist hat and listened to all the conversations that were going on around me with the staff. It was handover time as staff changed from night shift to day shift. It soon became apparent that at least two of the day staff were agency nurses and, for both, it was their first time in A&E at the QEUH. The nurse in charge had to give them a quick orientation as well as hand out duties for them to do. From what the nurse in charge was saying, this was a regular, if not daily, occurrence. Nursing time was being lost, explaining where everything was and describing the department routine; throughout the morning, the agency nurses had to ask multiple questions. This, once again, puts both patients and staff at risk of iatrogenic disease as actual nursing time is lost. Macgill and Pringle reported that Scottish Health Boards saw overspends in their budgets by the end of December 2022. This was a real cause for concern as there were three months still to run before the end of the financial year. Ayrshire and Arran Health Board advised that their nursing budget alone had resulted in an overspend of £3.7m. Much of the overspending was due to payments made to private nursing agencies to cover staff shortages, "costing £1m in November" alone (Macgill and Pringle, 2023). The excess cost to NHS Scotland is understandable when one looks at the hourly and annual pay points for RGNs. For example, when working for NHS Scotland, a band 5 RGN has an annual salary of £28,407 with a net rate equating to £11.16 per hour. For those who join the NHSGGC nursing bank that annual salary rises to between

£30,229 - £37,664, depending on experience. For those who choose to join a private agency, the hourly rate can be up to £60.63 per hour.[13]

Those working within the hospitals are not alone in feeling stressed and having poor mental health. A study by Auth et al. (2022) examined 24 research papers which looked at mental health issues suffered by emergency service workers (ESW). Although the majority of the papers looked solely at paramedics, it is important to note that eight of the papers included police and firefighters. It was noted that "[s]uicide attempts by EWS are considerably more prevalent than the estimated rate of 0.5% in the general population" (Auth et al. 2022, p. 1). This shocking statistic is backed up by Mars et al., who found that "the risk of suicides amongst male paramedics in the UK was found to be 75% higher than the national average" (2020, p. 11). Both papers propose a few reasons as to why this may be the case, the first being the number of traumatic incidents ESWs are exposed to, leading to an increase in the number of paramedics suffering from post-traumatic stress disorder (PTSD). Paramedics by the very nature of their work, are called to many traumatic incidents, something which can lead to PTSD, which, as Auth et al. note "increases suicidal risks" (2022, p. 2) within the emergency services. This correlates with the findings of Mars et al. who noted that "[t]here is growing evidence to suggest that ambulance staff may be at increased risk for suicide" (2020, p. 10). To combat such known risks, it is good working practice for those who have been called to a traumatic event to be offered a variety of programmes to prevent mental health issues. These include peer support systems, counselling, and a designated time for recovery. The availability and duration of these programs may differ from one health board to another, with some offering no recovery time and others allowing up to two hours (Halpern et al., 2009). When listening to Jordan's interview it was evident that having any sort of time out would be very problematic. With ambulance crews being held up in queues outside the hospital, there were fewer crews available to respond to calls, reducing that number by even one would not be possible with a service already stretched. The fact that iatrogenic disease in healthcare workers can lead to fatalities is a severe criticism of the NHS and the way it is managed.

What was anticipated was the second reason given for work stress, an increase in workload. With so much time being lost whilst crews are sitting in queues outside the QEUH, those still in service have to answer more calls, with the added pressure of being back on the road as soon as possible. Campbell

---

[13] Data for salaries can be found at: https://ambition24hours.co.uk/best-pay-rates-in-scotland#:~:text=Be%20one%20of%20the%20best,with%20%C2%A343.34%20per%20hour. https://apply.jobs.scot.nhs.uk/Job/JobDetail?jobid=161941&source=JobtrainRss https://www.net-paid.com/NHS-Hourly-Pay.php#:~:text=1st%20April%202024).-,NHS%20Band%204,before%20the%205%25%20NHS%20payrise..

quoted one paramedic as saying that the "[w]orkload is massive. You could have just dealt with a very complicated job and need a few minutes to gather your thoughts, but that time is never allowed as the control centre is constantly harassing you." (2022). It becomes a vicious circle as more paramedics take sick leave, those left behind have an increase in their workload, leading to increased stress, poor mental health, and more sick days. This increase in workload also relates to crews being unable to finish shifts on time when they are sitting waiting with patients in ambulance bays:

> purely from a selfish point of view, whilst we're doing all the waiting, you're not getting any break. Often, we're overdue our finish time because there's not enough of us to come and let us that are waiting get away. (Jordan, 2022).

The table below is constructed from the most recent data for the week beginning 8th July 2024. A turnaround time is calculated from the minute the ambulance arrives at the hospital until it is cleared to go back on the road. I have used hospitals from around the country, from cities, and towns to rural communities. I must point out that this period of time occurs during the Scottish school holidays and in particular, the Greenock Fair and the Aberdeen Trades holidays, with many people being away.[14]

**Figure 3.2** Ambulance Turnaround Times in Minutes for Week Beginning 8th July 2024.

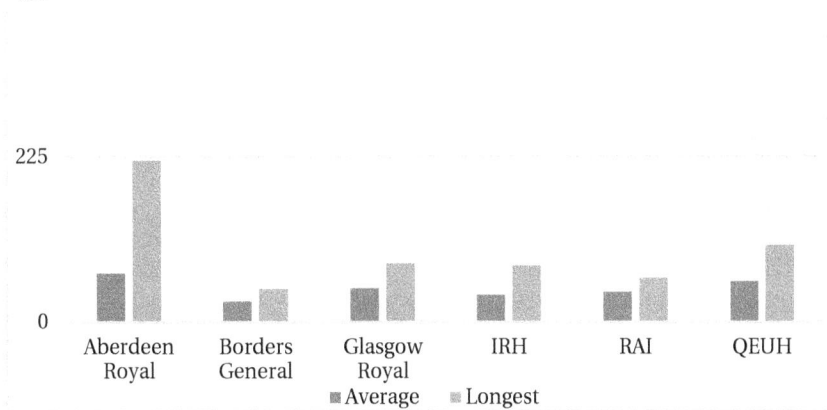

Data from the Scottish Ambulance Service. Available from: 2024 07 24 Weekly Operational Data (XLSX | 183KB), Table 7. Accessed: 30th July 2024.

---

[14] The Fair or Trades holidays were traditionally a two week holiday where the shipbuilding yards would close down. Each town and city would have a different two weeks with Glasgow following Greenock. Many local people still take their holidays during these two weeks.

A major concern voiced by Jordan would be if, as has been proposed, the IRH and the RAI were to close, all those ambulances would then be sent to the QEUH.

As mentioned in Chapter Two, Jordan suggested that the old Royal Hospital for Sick Children, Yorkhill, could be made into a specialised A&E hospital, thus increasing the number of ambulance bays available within the NHSGGC catchment area. At present, it operates as an outpatient clinic and diagnostic hub. In the early 1990s, the Health Department, in a bid to reduce A&E usage, established minor injury units. The first such unit in Scotland was opened at the Western General Hospital, Edinburgh, in 1994. These are now a nationwide common resource, either as stand-alone facilities, such as the one at the New Victoria Hospital or are attached to large A&E departments, with one being situated at the QEUH. McCarthy (2020) carried out research into the usage of minor injury units. Although waiting times in the units are shorter, as no complex medical cases or emergencies are seen there, people are still choosing to bypass such units and go instead to A&E with medical issues that do not require emergency treatment.[15] McCarthy noted that the younger the age, the more likely the individual was to go to A&E, "people aged 18-34 years were more than twice as likely to attend ED [Emergency Department] with a non-urgent condition, such as a minor injury, compared with other age groups" (2020, p.112). Although younger people accepted that waiting times were longer, they preferred to be seen by a doctor. The reasons behind such choices could be down to a lack of understanding as to the role of minor injury units and the skill levels of the emergency nurse practitioners. McCarthy also suggested that it could be because "successive governments have supported service users to view themselves as consumers of healthcare services rather than passive recipients, resulting in a stronger consumer culture within the NHS" (2020, p. 113). The government is attempting to shift people's perception of A&E departments as being the panacea for all ailments and has launched an advertising campaign signposting people to other healthcare services such as their local pharmacy or GP. McCarthy proposed that all such campaigns should be extended to include all social network platforms.

Finally, Auth et al. report that one-third of paramedics "experience mental health stigma, a rate that is higher than the general population" (2022, p. 2). As frontline staff, we rely on paramedics to be strong, confident, and professional in the case of an emergency, there may be added pressure to live up to this stereotype. It could be attributed to the fact that a significant number of

---

[15] Minor injury units have different opening hours and not all are staffed seven days a week. It must also be noted that McCarthy's research did not include NHS Scotland. Although minor injury units in other areas are walk in, to be granted access in Scotland you must first contact NHS111.

paramedics are male and that reporting mental health difficulties can be perceived as weakness, with macho culture preventing men from asking for help. The stigma associated with mental health, where individuals are judged negatively because of their mental or physical traits, can result in various forms of discrimination, whether overt or subtle. Goffman (1963) maintained that stigma exists through socially constructed norms, and, for some, the anticipation of perceived stigma may prevent an individual from actively seeking help. Halpern et al. found that "an organizational culture that stigmatizes vulnerability is the most insidious and challenging barrier to accessing support after a critical incident. Addressing the issue of stigma is critical to developing appropriate interventions." (2009, p. 139). Many diagnosed with mental illness experience a sense of shame brought about by a perceived feeling of being stigmatised. The pressure not to be shamed as being either weak or work-shy results in many paramedics working whilst mentally unwell.

When looking at the research surrounding stigma and shaming, I was reminded that shame is an emotion that is used to regulate behaviour and ensure compliance. Scheff writes that "shame is our moral gyroscope" (2003, p. 18). It is an emotion that not only regulates our future actions but also threatens the social bond of our relationships. Working relationships are crucial for ambulance crews as they work in pairs and rely heavily on each other, especially after traumatic callouts. One emotion that is a result of feeling shame is anger. This emotion bears an affinity with shame, with Scheff recognising that "one way of hiding shame is to become angry" (2003, p. 11). This anger can take various forms, directed both outwardly and inwardly. Among paramedics, this may result in frustration over losing the autonomy to decide when to take a break, complete a shift on schedule, or take time off after a distressing call. Then there is the anger they may feel at complying, at not questioning those situations, and never disputing the excess workload. Shame threatens the social bond and can bring about feelings of rejection and conflict. The fear of being seen as weak and the perceived threat to the social-workplace bond must be heightened when one takes into consideration that paramedics work in pairs.

The issue of women being critical of other women within the workplace is examined by Mavin et al. 2014 and Sheppard and Aquino, 2017, and I believe that this is pertinent across genders. Sheppard and Aquino's research pointed out that "there are consistent social penalties when women violate prescriptive stereotypes by behaving agentically" (2017, p. 696). With men, there are also social penalties with any deviation from the macho *stiff upper lip* of British culture being "perceived as a weakness.... unable to cope with the demands of the job" (Auth et al. 2022, p. 9). Through their work on hegemonic masculinities, Connell and Messerschmidt point out that "gender is always relational" (2005, p. 848) and gender patterns are socially defined in relation to masculinity or femininity. The stigma of weakness removing the social construct of strong masculinity may be too much to bear for some, resulting in either leaving the job or, sadly for a minority, suicide.

To combat mental health issues suffered by NHS England staff during the pandemic, the government set up 40 mental health hubs across the country. These were established to help alleviate feelings of stress and burnout among staff, they were there to help keep people healthy and, therefore, in work. Webber (2024) wrote of the success of the units, noting that "95% of the health workers treated at one hub returned to work or did not take sick absence". When the effectiveness of another hub was reviewed, data revealed that over 200 staff with long-term sickness had, in fact, returned to work. Sadly, despite excellent results from the hubs, since March 2023, 18 of the hubs have closed due to a slash in governmental funding from £38.5m in 2021 to only £2.3m in 2023. This appears to be a false economy as "for every £1 spent on workplace mental health interventions, £5 is saved" (Webber, 2024). With over £12 billion being spent by the NHS on sickness absences per year, many of which are through mental health issues, £38.5m seems to be money worth spent (Webber, 2024).[16]

Jake Jones, in his autobiography about his life as a paramedic, writes about the health problems he and, many of his colleagues, suffer. Many paramedics experience physical problems, from lifting patients and equipment to knee problems due to long periods of kneeling while performing cardiopulmonary resuscitation (CPR). However, there are still unseen mental health issues that affect many paramedics. He discusses the toll from shift work, a feeling of "permanent jet lag" (2020, p. 256), and the problems after witnessing so many traumatic incidents: grief, resentment, bitterness, addiction and relationship breakdowns. He writes, "[f]or some, in work terms, these problems are the final straw, for others, they might be the beginning of the end" (2020, p. 256), yet all paramedics, if they continue in the profession until retirement age (65 years for women and 67 years for men), are expected to still be carrying out the same physical tasks as a colleague 30 years their junior. This is surely not realistic.

The problems experienced by the ambulance services can also be attributed to a misuse of the service by the UK public. As Campbell reported, "[o]ver half of paramedics are suffering from burnout caused by overwhelming workloads, record numbers of 999 calls and the public misusing the ambulance service" (2022, p. 1). There is a nationwide problem of ambulances being called out to non-emergencies. One TikTok user wrote to tell me that they had reviewed ambulance waiting times as part of their MA dissertation, and the biggest

---

[16] NHSGGC has a staff mental health wellbeing system, but contact is virtual, see: https://www.nhsggc.scot/staff-recruitment/staff-support-and-wellbeing/.

reason for long waits was people using ambulances like a taxi service (TikTok user, 2022).

The enduring problem of ambulance callouts to non-emergency calls is one of the biggest problems to beset the ambulance service. (Jones, 2020). All 999 calls to the ambulance service are triaged and fall into one of four categories:

- Category 1: a threat to life, e.g., cardiac arrest; recommended response time of seven minutes.

- Category 2: serious condition but not an immediate threat to life, e.g., stroke; recommended response time 18 minutes.

- Category 3: urgent calls, e.g., abdominal pains; recommended response time of 120 minutes.

- Category 4: non-urgent calls, e.g., vomiting; referred to another service but if the patient insists on an ambulance, then recommended response time of 180 minutes. (Hall, 2022).

The first two categories necessitate an ambulance being sent, and the patient being transported to the hospital, patients in the third category can be treated at home by a medical practitioner, but not necessarily in a hospital. The fourth category does not require an ambulance to be sent or for the patient to be taken to the hospital. Patients that fall under category four are signposted to other services such as NHS 24 or their GP. The problems arise not with the first two categories but with the third and fourth categories and it is these that make up the majority of ambulance call-outs (Jones, 2020). This is consistent with data obtained by Hammett, who noted that "[a] recent study analysing 300 consecutive calls to the NHS found just over half – 54% – of the patients legitimately needed an ambulance" (2023, p. 1).

One problem that affects the NHS, nationwide, is the frequent callers, these patients not only take up ambulance time but are a financial drain on the ambulance service. Snooks et al. carried out research into the problem of frequent callers and sent questionnaires to 13 ambulance services; receiving replies from 12. They used the agreed, ambulance service, definition of a frequent caller as someone who makes over 12 calls in three months or five or more calls in a month. These callers make up a minority of all patients. However, when analysing the data received from the London Ambulance Service, Snooks et al. noted that in the period 2014–2015 out of the 1.7 million 999 calls received, 49,534 calls generated an ambulance attendance, with these attendance calls being made by only 1622 people. This cost to the London Ambulance Service was "£4.4 million" (2019, p. 2). The reason why they generate such high attendance rates is because they understand how the system works. They have acquired knowledge on how to beat the algorithm, knowing that if they complain of chest pain, they will be placed in category 1 or 2, necessitating an ambulance call out and a potential hospital visit (Jones, 2020).

With such high costs to Ambulance Services' resources and budgets, the NHS and the ambulance services must gain an understanding of the motivations behind frequent callers. One important factor that emerged from Snooks et al.'s research was the social demographic of these patients. They reported that not only was loneliness and vulnerability a common feature, but these callers were often "living in poverty and experiencing a lower quality of life than the general population" (2019, p. 2). They also noted that people tended to call 999 when they were experiencing a crisis or during a period of change, such as having just been discharged from a hospital or prison or a breakup of a relationship. All who fell into the frequent caller category had complex needs which were exacerbated during evenings and weekends. Despite being furnished with data that identified the characteristics of a frequent caller, with limited funds, and an unforeseen pandemic, no protocols have been put in place to deal with the problem (Snooks et al. 2019).

It is not just a misuse of ambulance services that is causing problems within the A&E departments of UK hospitals. A large majority of visits to A&E departments are for ailments that could be treated by a visit to a GP or a pharmacist. Research in 2018 revealed that the number of people who should have visited their GP instead of A&E was a staggering 20%. Despite having access to the NHS 24 free helpline, "[a} survey revealed that 1 in 3 admitted to attending A&E, simply because they were worried and didn't know what to do" (Hammett, 2023). Perhaps one way to tackle service misuse is to charge/fine those who call out ambulances or turn up at A&E with negligible complaints. In 2018 it was reported that there were 22,000 such complaints ranging from hangovers to splinters, to paper cuts (Hammett, 2023). Perhaps if it was made known that the costs to the NHS would be passed on to the patient it may act as a deterrent. The costs are:

- Each 999 ambulance call costs £7
- An ambulance dispatch costs £180
- An A&E visit by ambulance costs £233 (Hammett, 2023).

Nevertheless, for the frequent callers, not only would many be unable to meet the cost of any fine, but no financial consequence would be a deterrent due to their complex mental health and social needs.

Paramedics are increasingly coming under attack from those they are sent to help. From verbal to physical abuse, there has been an increase, year on year, of reported incidents. In the year 2020-2021 (the most recent data held), it was recorded that 11,749 crew members were abused or attacked. To put this into perspective, that is 32 incidents every day or "more than one every hour.... An increase of 4,060 incidents over the last five years" (AACE, 2023). In an attempt to reverse this trend, the Association of Ambulance Chief Executives (AACE) have launched *Work Without Fear*, a national campaign that aims to highlight the abuse suffered by ambulance crews and to foster an environment of respect for front-line emergency workers.

Fining those who misuse the NHS is not a new proposal. To counter the problem of missed GP appointments, it was suggested that a £10 fine be given to all those who miss appointments. NHS England reported that, in 2018, there were over 15 million missed GP appointments, which cost the NHS around £216 million.[17] If those appointments had not been made, the money saved could have been used for 58,320 hip replacement operations or 216,000 Alzheimer's drug treatments (NHS England, 2019). Research has been carried out into the reasons behind missed appointments and the results have shown a discrepancy across social demographic fields, with the number one identifying feature being "social deprivation" (BJGP, 2022). McQueenie et al. (2019) found similar results when carrying out research in Scotland. They noted a link between lower social class, chronic long-term conditions, poor mental health, and repeated missed appointments. A one-size-fits-all approach would have limited effects on the problem due to the complex needs of the patients. McQueenie et al. also found a link between repeated missed appointments and "premature all-cause mortality rates" (2019, p. 8). Missed appointments mean that medication and treatment plans cannot be reviewed, or new problems identified. Many missed appointments also resulted in a deterioration in health and a 999 call-out. One solution that has been suggested has been to give those, who repeatedly miss appointments an on-the-day consultation (BJGP, 2022; McQueenie et al., 2019).

It has been over a decade since the British coalition government began its austerity programme. Despite many of the country's public services seeing their budgets slashed, the NHS was protected from cuts. Yet, despite small increases year on year to the NHS, when one takes into account inflation and the increased financial burden on the service:

- An increasing elderly demographic, the cost of medical care for the elderly is "from three to four times higher than for people under 50" (Leys, 2020)
- An increase in people living in poverty
- New medical discoveries and treatments
- Governmental loans to cover shortfalls in budgets

---

[17] Each GP visit costs £30 and lasts 15 minutes.

- Repairs and maintenance to hospital buildings resulting in a "backlog of £ 6 billion in repairs" (Leys, 2020)

- Payments to private agencies to cover staff shortages.

Add to this cuts to the numbers of community nurses and NHS dentists led to greater pressure being placed on GP surgeries, and, when people failed to get appointments, they would turn to A&E. The austerity programme has, inadvertently, placed more pressure on the NHS.

The BMA reported striking statistics in their 2022 report titled *The Country is Getting Sicker.* It goes without argument that poverty kills, and with the austerity programme and today's economic crisis, it is not surprising to see numbers living in poverty rising. Food and fuel poverty are major contributing factors to ill health "cold homes are associated with reduced resistance to respiratory infections" (BMA, 2022). It is estimated that the cost to the NHS, through treatment of those suffering from illnesses directly linked to cold, damp homes, was £2.5billion in 2021. The BMA also reported that '[i]n September 2022, 18% (9.7 million adults) of all households were food insecure" (BMA, 2022). This number has more than doubled since January of the same year. The result is that people are unable to provide good quality healthy foods, such as fruit and vegetables. What was particularly marked was that 4.8 million people do not own kitchen appliances such as a cooker or a fridge. Living without a fridge or a freezer means that a person has to shop everyday as they cannot keep fresh food. For those who find themselves in this situation it has been estimated that there is a 43% increase in their food bills, around "£1,365 a year to an average family" (BMA, 2022).

At the beginning of this chapter, I posed McLardy-Smith's question "The NHS as an employer is it worth saving?" (2022, p. 31). Despite the many problems highlighted in this chapter, I believe it is, but that will require a lot of reform. As it is such a large topic it requires more than just a few sentences. As a result, in the concluding of this book, Dr Stead will propose suggestions that have been put forward by staff, past and present, researchers, politicians and health consultants. Proposals that may help with the issues discussed in this chapter. Suggestions that may help mend NHS Scotland and take it out of critical care, restoring it to its former glory. There is no easy fix to decades of failings, and social reform will be necessary. However, will any government be brave enough to tackle the problems head-on and attempt to reform this institution?[18] The Scottish general public may not be open to change.

---

[18] On the 22nd May 2024 the then British Prime Minister, Rishi Sunak, called a General Election with the NHS being a major political battleground. The subsequent electoral result on the 4th July 2024 saw an overwhelming majority for the Labour Party with Keir Stammer becoming Prime Minister.

# Chapter Four
# An Unequal Health Service

## Yvonne Bennett

Health care should be provided equally to everyone regardless of background, ability, and lifestyle. In this chapter, we investigate age-related disparities in healthcare services highlighted by participants. The daughters of Ella, Jean, and John all shared similar traumatic experiences whilst their elderly parents were receiving health care at the QEUH. All three were admitted to the hospital after being brought to the A&E department, having been assessed by paramedics and needing further medical care. In subsequent chapters, we will analyse data obtained from semi-structured interviews, social media content, and private messages. At this juncture, we wish to briefly outline what each family experienced to allow for context. The following section of data is anecdotal which we recognise can make it problematic as it has limitations being as it is based on memory. Individuals are subjective, and as such, we do not assert that the following narratives are historically unbiased. As Maines, Pierce, and Laslett remind us, "individuals make history under conditions not of their own making" (2008, p. 44); our participants' experiences are entwined in the societal conditions of the time. However, we argue that this data is both empirical and verifiable due to the nature of the subject under investigation. Case notes, and content on media, both social and traditional, may be used to ratify the following narratives.

### A Synopsis of Experience

My mum, **Ella,** was convalescing in a care home in Glasgow. She had become ill in February 2022 and had been admitted to the Inverclyde Royal Hospital (IRH). Until this time, she cared, full-time for my dad, Sandy, who had contracted long COVID. As a result of her illness, both parents had to move into a care home, where my dad died on May 2nd 2022. On Tuesday, 10th August 2022, the day of my mother's accident, my brother and I treated her to dinner. The following day, I had planned to take her shopping to find an outfit for my eldest son's upcoming wedding, which was just a few weeks away. I had returned to my daughter's flat and received a phone call from the care home charge nurse around 8.30 pm saying that my mum had had a fall. He suspected she had fractured her femur, and they were waiting for the ambulance. It was agreed that I would meet the ambulance at A&E as I was closer to the hospital than the care home. My mum lay on the floor of the care home for five hours before a first responder arrived and was able to give some pain relief.[1] He assessed that an ambulance was required, and the paramedics arrived around twenty minutes later and were able to administer some pain relief, although it helped, it did not fully control her pain. When I met the ambulance at the QEUH we had to wait a further hour, outside, in a queue of ambulances before my mum could be admitted. My mum's distress and pain will live with me. She was too frail to use the Entonox machine.[2] The paramedics were frustrated by their inability to help. When she was eventually admitted it was ten hours from the accident until she was given a nerve block and was finally pain-free. Throughout this period, she was extremely confused and frightened, my mum, up until this point had always been *as sharp as a tack*.

I was told they would only be able to operate that day if she had not been given her anti-coagulant drug the evening before, as it had to be out of her system for a minimum of 24 hours. A call to the care home ascertained that she had not had the drug. Unfortunately, due to theatre lists, the operation was postponed until the following day, despite having been in the hospital since around 2 am. The next morning, Thursday, the anaesthetist spoke to my brother to get consent to operate, which was to take place around 11 am. I also spoke to the ward nurse and was told that she was ready for theatre. Ten minutes later, the care home called me to say that the operation had been cancelled as her anti-coagulant had been administered, in error, by hospital staff the previous evening. I was aware, after a conversation with the orthopaedic doctor in A&E, that there was an optimum 72-hour window in which to perform the repair. We were told that the anaesthetist on rota that day would not perform the operation until the drug was 48 hours out of her system, given her age and frailty. The optimum window would have been closed by then.

After a consultant's meeting with the doctors and the orthopaedic nurse, it was agreed to carry out the operation the following morning. Although the operation was successful, my mum remained confused and failed, many times, to recognise either my brother or myself. We lost our mum in August 2022; she may not have died then but she never fully recovered from the trauma. The final seven months of her life, she lived with confusion and fear, barely recognizing us.

---

[1] A first responder is a volunteer who is trained to attend certain types of emergency calls in the area where they live or work. The aim is to have a medically trained individual arrive in the first vital minutes before the ambulance crew can arrive.

[2] Entonox is a mixture of nitrous oxide and oxygen. It is commonly called gas and air, or laughing gas, and is used during labour.

**Jean**, our mum, became unwell on 2nd November 2020. I took a call from her home caregiver telling me that Mum was finding it difficult to breathe. I called an ambulance and went to her house; she lived close by. The paramedics assessed her and said that she needed to go to A&E. Given her Alzheimer's diagnosis, I was allowed to accompany her, however, once we arrived at the QEUH, the nursing staff denied me access (as per COVID-19 protocol). I refused to stay outside and went into A&E; she needed me to advocate for her. The doctor diagnosed my mum with an exacerbation of her Chronic Obstructive Pulmonary Disease (COPD), and after getting her stabilised with oxygen, I was told to go home as she would be admitted to an acute medical ward. I tried over 40-50 times to call the ward that afternoon and evening, but no one answered the phone. The next morning, a doctor called me to say that she had been unsettled overnight, and they needed me to agree to a Do Not Resuscitate (DNR) order being set up; I refused. Despite being told that someone would call to update me during the day, no one did, and still, no one answered the phone. I eventually got through to the ward that evening and was told by a member of the nursing staff that she had deteriorated, not long afterwards, the consultant called and told me she was improving on antibiotics. I asked about her COVID test and was told that the results were not back, but that COVID was not a death sentence, with over 80% of people surviving. As a family, we felt reassured and were given a pass for one member of the family to go and visit. My brother agreed to go. He was shocked to see her still in a hospital gown despite having her nightwear with her. When he looked in the bedside cabinet, he found another patient's belongings despite the room having been deep cleaned [per infection control protocol]. As my brother was leaving, a nurse told him my mum was now positive for COVID. We were all extremely worried as not only did she have COPD, but she was also diabetic. As soon as I heard the news, I went to see her, she had not been washed, nor catheterised since being admitted almost 48 hours earlier.

The following morning a doctor called to say she had deteriorated, and they wanted the DNR to be signed. I refused and was asked to come to the ward. She had now been transferred to a COVID ward and when I got there, I found her slumped in bed, struggling to breathe with a fever. She had not had her medication. The doctors were insisting I sign the DNR, and when I once again refused was told they would take it out of my hands and put one in place. They told me she would not be ventilated, and they would not give her the anti-viral drug widely used by the NHS, at that time, to treat COVID. After I begged them, they agreed to start her on it via an intravenous (IV) drip. I sat with her all night, and, in the early hours of the morning, they prescribed Midazolam to keep her calm.[3] I went home to change and have a shower and when I got no answer to repeated phone calls, I went back. When I looked through the window in the door to my mum's room, I could see she was a strange colour. As I opened the door and walked in, I could hear the hiss from the oxygen machine, she had the mask on, but it wasn't connected to the tubing, she was dead.

I called for help, and everyone started running, I was taken to a room, and half an hour later, they came to tell me she had died. I screamed that they had killed her, they said it was an accident. Her death certificate says that she died of COVID. It wasn't COVID that killed her. It was the hospital. They had washed and changed her and didn't re-connect the tube. They are denying that and blaming my mum for disconnecting it, but her hands were deformed with severe osteoarthritis. She couldn't have disconnected the tube; she couldn't even do up her buttons. We fought for a post-mortem, but the Procurator Fiscal, after initially agreeing, changed his mind.[4] I will never get over walking into that room and finding my mum dead, I get comfort in that she would have passed peacefully in her sleep.

On Saturday, 23rd October 2021 my dad, **John,** suffered a heart attack. He was taken by ambulance to the Royal Alexandra Hospital (RAH) in Paisley. He was taken there because, despite being closer to the QEUH, his postcode had the RAH as his designated A&E hospital when being admitted by ambulance. On admission, he tested positive for COVID and was placed in a COVID ward, and further tests revealed he had three blocked arteries. He was told that the operation to fix these would be carried out at the Golden Jubilee private hospital as the NHS Scotland outsourced procedures to them to improve waiting lists. As he had tested positive for COVID, the operation could not be carried out immediately. He was discharged home after two days to await an outpatient appointment.

I called him on Friday, 29th October 2021, to check in and he surprised me by asking if I could come over. This request was out of character for my dad, who had always been incredibly independent. When I arrived, he was breathless. I tested him for COVID, the test was negative, and I administered his nebuliser.

---

[3] Midazolam is a widely used end-of-life sedative and controversy surrounds its use during the pandemic with its use in care homes doubling during the pandemic. Inquiries into this increase are now underway with some media sources calling its use as a euthanasia pathway.

[4] A procurator fiscal works for the Crown Office and decides if there is enough evidence to take a case to court. Any sudden, unexplained deaths are referred to the procurator fiscal and they decide if a post-mortem is required.

There was no improvement the following morning, and I called NHS 24 for advice.[5] I was advised to see if things settled down, and they called me back three hours later. As he hadn't improved, they requested an ambulance be sent out. We waited over six hours and when the paramedics arrived, they found his blood oxygen levels to be extremely low. He was taken by ambulance to the RAH. Nine hours later he called me to say he was coming home as he was still in the ambulance waiting in a queue to be seen. He was freezing when he got home as he only had a thin blanket to keep him warm, and, as per COVID protocol, the ambulance doors had to be kept open.

I stayed with him overnight, and he had a fall, I called an uncle for help, and we decided to take him by car to the QEUH. Before we left, I tested him again for COVID and the test was negative. When we arrived at A&E, we were put into a room that had a COVID Waiting Room on the door. I was worried as I hadn't had COVID, and my dad had just recovered from it. When I complained and explained the situation, I was told to leave the door open. As he was getting more breathless and distressed, we were admitted to an A&E bay. I was told my dad had COPD, which was a surprise, and they administered oxygen. I was watching and listening to all that was being said and done. I learnt that with COPD your oxygen levels must be between 88% and 92% and that the colour of the valve on the oxygen tubing regulates the flow of oxygen.[6] The nurses were concerned that his oxygen levels kept dipping and that we had to try to keep him as calm as possible. I was angry as we had been in the hospital for over 12 hours, and no one had even offered us a drink. I was then told he was being moved into resus (the resuscitation area) as a precaution. As I could see the medical staff working on other very sick patients, I went home.

The following morning, I called and was told he had pneumonia and another heart problem and had been admitted to the COVID section of the Coronary Care High Dependency Unit, there were to be no visitors. I explained that both his COVID tests that week had been negative. We were being told, at this point, that he was settled, had started eating and was making improvements. Finally, we were told that I and his ex-partner (they remained close friends) could visit as we were his next of kin. He was sitting up talking but seemed confused, and, as we were leaving, he told me he loved me, this was not something my dad had

---

[5] NHS 24 is Scotland's national telephone advice and triage service. It covers out of hours periods and is accessed by dialing 111 as opposed to the emergency line on 999.

[6] Low oxygen therapy is used for those with diseases such as COPD, advanced Cystic Fibrosis or lung scarring. In these patients, the target oxygen saturation levels are between 88-92%. To administer the oxygen at too fast a rate can cause the blood oxygen levels to rise above 92% leading to possible hypercapnic respiratory failure. This is when the body retains $CO_2$.

ever said. On Monday morning, I called and was told he had deteriorated and that we needed to have the family at the hospital. My stepsister had been estranged from my dad for over six years, but I called her. When she arrived at the ward, my dad became agitated and distressed and wanted her to leave. The medical staff decided to give him something to calm him down.[7] Myself and his ex-partner were allowed to stay for as long as we wanted.

I sat with him and noticed that the monitor was not recording his blood oxygen levels. I was shocked as I remembered all that I had heard in A&E. A nurse came in, and before I could say anything, she turned the monitor off saying, 'I feel you are looking at that all the time'. I was worried as I couldn't see his oxygen stats on the machine. I noticed that when I went out, his oxygen machine would be turned down when I came back in. I asked the nurse, and she said that I must have leant on it. It was a knob that turned it up and down, so I knew I hadn't done anything. We decided then that we would always have one of us with him.

The nurse in charge came in and told us that my stepsister had called and that he had told her to come up. I was angry as it had been written down how distressed my dad had been when he saw her. The nurse responded that it was her right to be informed, and if we had any issues with this decision, I should take it up with my stepsister directly. Then they brought in a machine that was a slow-release thing that gave the drug over 24 hours. It didn't seem to be working as before the 24 hours were up his fingertips were blue. When I queried it, they said it was because he was on low oxygen, yet they told me earlier he was on maximum. Then I noticed that his tubing had been changed, so it was the weakest one. They had also put on a mask, and we asked for the nose cannulas, but we were told that he didn't have long to go, so that was why they used the mask. They then said that they were going to take the mask off so we could say our goodbyes. He made a gasping sound and went black, pure black. They asked us to go out of the room so they could move him, but when we went back in, he was still in the same position. We will never know if they were turning down his oxygen or if he was on it at all, as I couldn't see the stats on the machine. Some things we will never know. He died a week after he was admitted, but he had been getting better.

John's death certificate states he died of COVID pneumonia, but his family disputes this. A few weeks later, the family received his out-patient's appointment for the Golden Jubilee Hospital, causing more distress.

---

[7] This may have been Midazolam, but we are unable to confirm or refute this.

**Image 3.1** The Wingate Family.

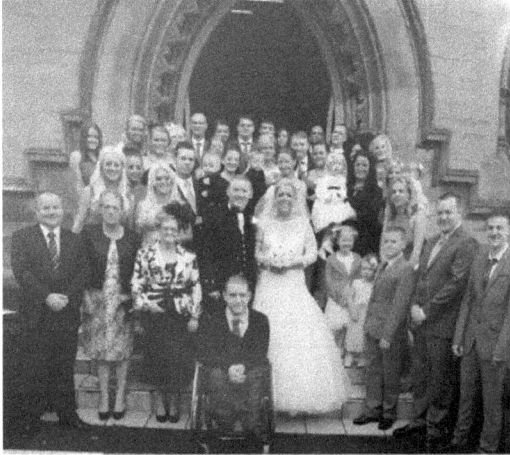

**Image 3.2** The Nimmo Family.

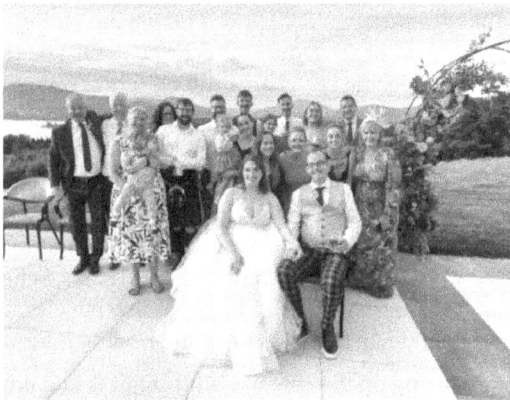

**Image 3.3** The Jackson Family.

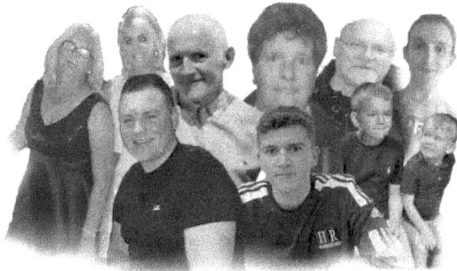

**Image 3.4** The Jackson Family.

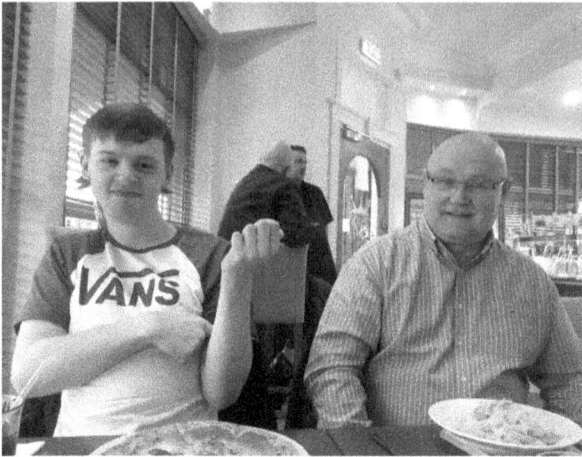

## Social Care at Home

As discussed in the introduction, Scotland is an ageing nation with a growing number of elderly. The role of the family in social care must be considered. This exploration will have a specific focus on adult children. Care for the elderly is achieved through one of two networks: formal, by medical practitioners or informal, by family, friends and neighbours. Progressively, it is the informal network that is being called upon as the primary support system. The provision of informal care can lead to an emotional shift in family relationships as we have to parent our parents. To date, various studies have examined the informal care networks in several countries (Mendes et al., 2018; Ris, Scnepp and Imhof, 2018; Andruske and O'Conner, 2020). These studies have examined cultural beliefs surrounding elderly care as well as the burden felt by informal caregivers.

Adult children are taking on the role of both caregiver and advocate, to their elderly parents, when it comes to navigating the health care system in Scotland. They take on these roles to ensure their parents receive care that is both adequate and dignified. This is not a new situation, four decades ago, Cierelli wrote that "[w]hen elderly people do feel the need for help, they prefer to receive it from their adult children above all others." (1981, p. 161) a sentiment that those of us who find ourselves belonging to the sandwich generation can relate to. With social care being squeezed through budget cuts, caregiving is pushed more and more into the informal network. This tends, as has traditionally been the case, to be a role that falls, unequivocally, onto women. Sherrell and Newton noted that "[t]he majority of middle-aged women with a surviving parent can expect to experience parental caregiving at some point" (1996, p. 175). In 2018, Mendes et al. carried out a study in Brazil into the physical, emotional, and social burdens informal caregivers can experience.

Their research findings correlated with Sherrell and Newton's results 22 years earlier, in that it was middle-aged women made up the majority of informal caregivers. Mendes et al. reported that the average age of a caregiver in Brazil was 53 years, with only 8.7% being male. It was noted that 55.3% of the care given was by an adult child (2018). Research shows a cultural element is present with different cultures presenting different data on the predominance of women undertaking the role. Research by Andruske and O'Connor (2018) looked at the experiences of immigrant communities within Canada. They discovered that Chinese women made up 78% of primary carers in their community, for the South Asian communities, it was 70% and 80% for those of Latin American heritage. This is in stark comparison when one considers that in the UK, that number is 59%, with male carers only slightly in the minority. (Age UK, 2018), a statistic I found to be surprising.

**Figure 4.1** Percentage of Carers Based on Gender.

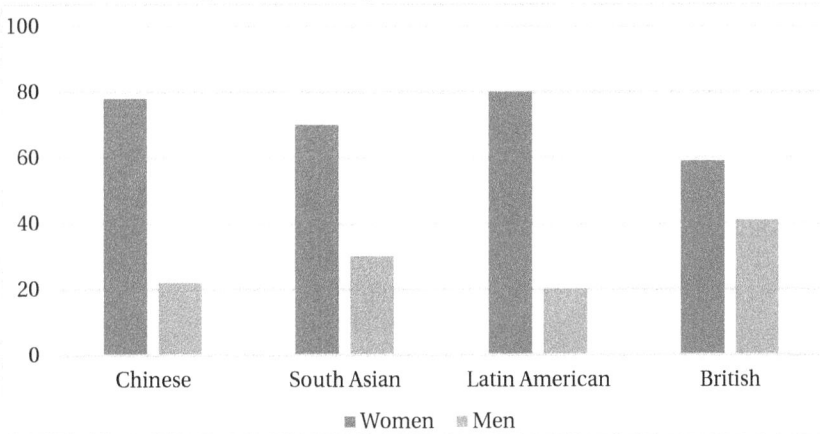

Data from: Andruske, C. L., and O'Connor, D. (2020) "Family care across diverse cultures: Re-envisioning using a transnational lens." *Journal of Aging Studies*, volume, 55, pp. 1 – 10.

Interestingly, Andruske and O'Connor did report that, within the immigrant communities, there is a difference in expectations between first and second-generation immigrants. Those, who are at present the caregiver, expressed a desire that this role would not fall on their children when it came to their care. They noted a change in values, from the embedded cultural values of their parents to the Canadian values of their adopted homeland. One participant was quoted as saying, "I am Canadian now, the day that I begin to fail, in front of my house, there is a nursing home, you don't have to do any more than cross the street, and you can put me there." (2018, p. 5).

Varying expectations parents have for their children can lead to resentment. This resentment may be aimed at both siblings, seen as not doing their fair share and at the parents themselves. My parents expected that I would be the one to help as my brother was 'too busy with work', I was undertaking a PhD at the time and lived over five hundred miles away. Any help my brother did give, or when he visited, was greeted with such adoration. Luckily, my brother was aware of the situation, and there were many humorous conversations about his *golden child* status. If he did offer to help, it would often be rejected as not needed, and then they would call me. This is a situation many of my female friends find themselves dealing with. This expectation brought to the fore the question; why does this differing of expectation exist when it comes to gender? Is it because women are perceived as being more nurturing or as traditionally being the caregiver, taking on this role from children through to elderly parents? If the root cause is indeed differing gender expectations related to traditional roles, is it possible that over time, there could be a shift as parents become more conscious of raising children in a gender-neutral way? This gap in scholarship requires more investigation.

Taking on the role of caregiver is complicated, Sherrell and Newton posed the question, "[c]ould it be that the term 'role-reversal' has negative connotations for ageing, and it is too simplistic a way of looking at the complex interpersonal relationships that occur when one looks after an elderly parent?" (1996, p. 175). Caring for one's parents can heighten emotions and change family relationships, be that for the better or worse. Sherrell and Newton propose that when taking on the role of caregiver, one should then re-negotiate the relationship with parents, and by doing so, one "solidifies their own adult identity" (1996, p. 175). This is easier said than done. My dad was extremely independent, and to lose control over aspects of his life was devastating. On the few times that I voiced my concerns my dad would become angry and my mum tearful. There was no negotiation to be had. I was still their child and, as such, was to respect their decisions without argument. What took me by surprise, though, was to suddenly confront my own ageing and mortality. At this point, only two aunts remain between myself and my husband Graeme as the senior generation in our family. This realisation is what has solidified my adult identity.

Both Roseanne and Tracey's parents still lived alone at home. Roseanne took on the role of caregiver to her mum, a role she shared with her brother. Roseanne saw her role as a caregiver as one that was a natural progression "it was my turn to look after her". The family had also organised two home caregivers to go in every day to make sure she had taken her medication, prepared meals and did light household chores. Roseanne visited daily. Tracy realised her dad was extremely unwell when he asked her to come and stay with him. This was a role Tracy had not envisaged having to do, as her dad had been fiercely independent. Keeping their parents safe at home during the pandemic was paramount to Roseanne and Tracy. The UK media, during the first wave of COVID-19, portrayed it as a certain death sentence for the elderly:

- We were trying to keep her safe, speaking to her through windows, we got her wee garden done up so we could sit in the garden with her. (Roseanne, 2022)

- My dad was the safest most [sic] safest person ever, like he had gloves in his car, he had masks in his car, he had sanitiser. (Tracy, 2022).

Looking after an elderly parent at home can be costly: physically, emotionally, and financially. The emotional toll was heightened during the pandemic as fear surrounding the safety of the elderly was a constant. Daily television broadcasts from the First Minister, Nicola Sturgeon, gave numbers of deaths with demographic breakdowns.[8] These daily, one-hour broadcasts lasted for over a year, long after the UK-wide broadcasts had stopped.

The Scottish Government provides free care for all elderly over the age of 65 years who require assistance. This is either free personal care (FPC), help with personal hygiene, assistance at mealtimes and help with mobility, or free personal nursing care (FPNC), where care is required to be supervised by a trained nurse. This care can be provided at home or in a residential care home. The table below shows how much, in £ millions, this has cost the Scottish Government in 2011 and again in 2020.

**Figure 4.2** Cost to the Scottish Government for Free Elderly Care.

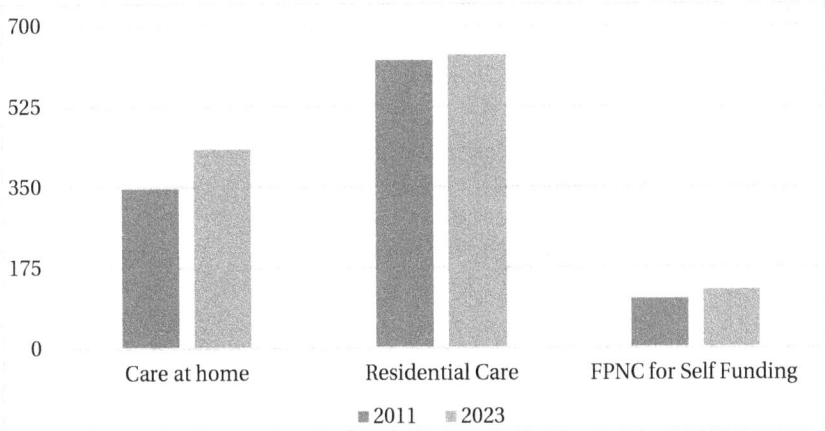

Data from: Scottish Government (2022) *Free Personal and Social Nursing Care, Scotland, 2020 – 2021*. Available at: https://www.gov.scot/publications/free-personal-nursing-care-scotland-2020-21/pages/3/. Accessed: 31st October 2023.

---

[8] The First Minister is the head of the Scottish Government and is accountable to the Scottish Parliament.

As can be seen, the costs are rising and set to rise further. With Scotland's changing age demographic, the burden of this cost will fall on fewer and fewer taxpayers.

The majority of elderly who receive either FPC or FPNC are cared for at home. The Scottish Government estimates that there are around 700,000 unpaid carers throughout the nation, receiving an average of 9.8 hours of paid help per week. The annual cost to the government, if these carers were to be paid, would be around £36 billion. To put this in perspective, the total annual budget for NHS Scotland is £13.4 billion (Scottish Government, 2022). For those who can no longer be cared for at home, there are local authority-run care homes. These provide care at a reduced rate and are means-tested. As of March 2022, there were 1051 registered care homes in Scotland of which only 11% were local authority owned. The average cost, per week, in a privately run care home for those needing personal care is £1341, if nursing care is required the cost rises to £1443 per week. The Scottish Government's free care subsidies contribute a maximum of £233.10 for FPC and an additional £104.90 if FPNC is also needed (Care Information Scotland, 2023). The reality is that for many, self-funded residential care is financially out of their reach. For those who are in residential care, the Scottish Government shoulders the cost of the care when the elderly person has £20,250 left in savings. I must add that this amount includes all assets, meaning that any property must have been sold and the proceeds already used. Taking this into account, plus the shortage of local authority-run homes it is of no surprise that the number of those being cared for, at home by unpaid carers, is so high.

It is not only a financial burden that is placed on informal caregivers, but it can also "generate physical, psychological, and social isolation" (Mendes et al., 2018). The physical demands of administering care may contribute to the physical fatigue experienced by those giving care on a daily basis. This is especially problematic if the caregiver is elderly or in poor physical health. Mendes et al.'s Brazilian research discovered that the carers who experienced the highest burden were the spouses; bound, perhaps, by their marriage vow of "in sickness and in health" (2018, p. 91). Caregiving changes not only the relationship with the elderly relative but can also lead to a decline in one's mental health as their own life undergoes significant changes. For example, social isolation, having to give up work, and a change in the relationship, all take a toll on mental health. Yet, Ris, Schnepp and Imhof argue that caregivers "may also benefit from the act of caregiving and that caregiving can be a rewarding experience" (2018, p. 96). For all who care for elderly relatives at home, we should try to remember that "to choose to include the elderly in our lives is to affirm not only their value but our own" (Koch, 1990, p. 212). We may not always feel appreciated for all we do, and we may, at times, lack patience as we attempt to parent our parents, it is a new path that we tread.

When we finally persuaded our parents to have daily paid care in January 2022, it was suggested, by the care company, that we use a male carer as my dad could relate to him better. This proved to be the case, and they both thought that the male carer, Robert, was wonderful.[9] What we hadn't realised, until our mum was admitted to hospital, and we had to stay with dad, was that our mum was getting up an hour earlier to make sure our dad was all ready for Robert, there was little for him to do. This was not the case when, on Robert's days off, a female carer would be sent. This may have been caused by the aforementioned stereotypical perception that caregivers are women, and they did not see Robert in that role. They saw him as someone who would help with heavier tasks, like moving my dad's oxygen machine or helping with an IT problem. When looking at the literature surrounding caregivers, be they paid or not, the overriding findings were that this was a job that women still found themselves undertaking. Once again, this may simply be down to traditional gender-assigned roles, with women being seen as more compassionate or more capable.

Amarante noted that within the private care at-home sector, "just over 18% of the workforce is male" (July 2023, blog). With so many job vacancies within the industry, some companies are targeting young male school leavers, hoping to change the gender imbalance (Amarante, 2023). By carrying out recruitment drives in schools and colleges, making young men aware of what a career in the sector entails could help to address the gender imbalance across the sector. This correction of the gender imbalance has also been found to benefit the care companies: "[a] survey by Business in the Community found that 90% of employers that take a more inclusive approach to their recruitment and workforce have said that they have higher skill levels, enhanced reputation and improve staff morale" (Amarante, 2023). My mum's care home had taken steps to address the gender imbalance, with around 30% of the staff being male; from the charge nurses, to care assistants and the catering staff. Gender diversity surrounds our lives when we are independent, it should not change as we require help.

### NHS Scotland: Care of the Elderly

The emphasis on elderly care within a hospital setting should focus on maintaining the dignity and the autonomy of the patient, yet our data reveals that this is not happening across all settings. Koch wrote that "[a]ge is not a firm line" (1990, p.211); the elderly are not a single entity to be treated as a *class* but are

---

[9] Robert is a pseudonym.

individuals with diverse life experiences. Nonetheless, research shows that in many cases, the elderly are being treated as one homogenous group (Lothian and Philp, 2001). Age does not come alone and is often debilitating; this can be both frustrating and frightening when faced with hospital admission. It is important that the elderly patient, and their family, receive adequate information to enable them to make choices to maintain a sense of autonomy. This is assisted by proper nursing assessment and care, taking into account the six core values of nursing: care, compassion, competence, communication, courage, and commitment (Ellis and Standing, 2023).

When I began this research project, much was written about patient-centred care (PCC). The overall premise is, that from the start of any medical intervention, a fundamental good quality of care could be achieved by utilising PCC. This collaborative model is deemed crucial for patient care as it treats patients as individuals and equal partners thus emphasising patient autonomy. The medical practitioner should furnish the patient with all the relevant information to enable them to make their own health and care path decisions. Assessments should be carried out holistically, taking into consideration the patient's "mental, physical, cognitive, behavioural, social and spiritual needs" (Ellis and Standing, 2023, p. 4). However, recent research by Alison Pilnick argues that it is difficult to accurately assess how effective PCC is. She puts forward that as PCC was introduced in the 1950s as a means of modernising patient care, it is now "framed as morally imperative" (2023, p. 1). Its moral aspect makes it difficult to critique. Although many research studies have looked at specific aspects of PCC, Pilnick points out that there are only three reviews of PCC as a whole, all of which find it to be lacking when it comes to overall changes in patients' health behaviours and outcomes. Pilnick's study was extensive as she looked at 25 years of video recordings of health practitioner-patient interactions. Her final findings suggested that theoretical approaches involving active patient participation in practitioner-patient interactions may seem effective in theory, but they may not consistently translate into practical success. She also made an interesting observation that "PCC, through the use of specific discursive practices, constitutes an ideal patient with particular kinds of intellectual and interactional attributes" (2023, p. 3).

Her conclusions lead to two issues: these being with authority and knowledge. These issues can further be divided into;

- Epistemic authority: the power over knowledge,
- Deontic authority: the power accorded by holding that knowledge.

If a doctor perceives that they hold both power and knowledge in a patient-doctor interaction, then PCC is only ever afforded lip service.

Pilnick's findings are supported by research that has revealed that the elderly do not always receive appropriate consideration and care (Lothian and Philp, 2001; Carvalho dos Santos and Ceolim, 2007; Singh and Okeke, 2016; Ben-Harush et al., 2007). According to Carvalho dos Santos and Ceolim, elderly patients "are generally treated as regular adult patients, without considering the singularity of the senescence and senility process" (2007, p. 809). The result of such treatment is an increased risk for iatrogenic injury. In a recent article, Permpongkosol looked at the risk elderly people face from iatrogenic disease during hospital admissions. This may be due, in part, to their increased core morbidities and, as a result, they require more medication. Permpongkosol identified that an increase in medications can lead to drug-induced iatrogenic disease which "transforms the elderly into living 'chemistry sets'" (2022, p.78). Several iatrogenic incidents can occur due to being prescribed a large cocktail of medications. One such incident is the pharmaceutical risk of certain medications counteracting with others. Other iatrogenic cases can be down to nursing errors: forgetting to give certain drugs at specific times, administering the wrong dosage or concentration of a drug, administering the drug by the wrong route (e.g., intravenously as opposed to intra-muscular), and even giving the medication to the wrong patient. See Chapter Five.

One concern that has arisen since the pandemic has been the perceived overprescribing, to the elderly, of the sedative Midazolam.[10] Both Roseanne and Tracy believe that their parents were given the drug. Reports in the mainstream UK media noted in 2020 that "[o]fficial figures show out-of-hospital prescribing of the drug midazolam increased by more than 100% in April compared to previous months." (Adams and Bancroft, 2020). These figures are the number of community prescriptions issued for the elderly being cared for in care homes and at home. The difficulty one has with these figures is that this sudden increase corresponded with the UK peak of overall deaths. Therefore, it is impossible to ascertain if the deaths were caused by the use of Midazolam or if Midazolam was prescribed to manage symptoms as part of an end-of-life pathway. The stories in the UK media are factually correct when it comes to numeral data but the cause of such a rise has not, and I would argue, cannot be verified.

When the elderly are admitted to a hospital, they tend to require more nursing care with hospital stays often being longer than younger patients. I had to advocate for my mum to have her discharged back to her care home. By doing so, we were able to prevent iatrogenic injury. This was something we had not been able to do on a previous hospital admission to the IRH when she

---

[10] Midazolam is a sedative given by injection. It is used to relieve anxiety pre surgery or medical procedures. It is also used within anesthesia. It belongs to the benzodiazepine group of medicines.

developed a pressure sore, "a frequent iatrogenic event" (Carvalho dos Santos and Ceolim, 2009, p. 809). There are also concerns that on discharge from the hospital, there is a failure to adequately meet the needs of the elderly, especially those with dementia who can no longer self-advocate. Much of this is caused by inadequate discharge documentation, which then prevents a smooth hospital-to-care/home transition (Parker et al. 2021). However, not all patients can be discharged causing an increase in cost to NHS Scotland, not only through the financial cost of caring for the individual but through the use of private hospitals to reduce waiting lists.

Delayed discharge patients, or *bed blockers*, are a major contributing factor when it comes to long waiting lists. The Scottish Government carries out a monthly and annual census to determine the number of patients awaiting discharge and the amount of time they have been waiting. The latest annual census, to the end of March 2023, reveals that there were 18,157 patients on delayed discharge for the financial year 2022-2023. These delays resulted in beds being blocked for a total of 661,705 days. The average amount of time the discharge was delayed was 11 days, but interestingly, the average stay of each patient before the delay was 44 days, making the average hospital stay a total of 55 days. The reasons behind the delays were varied but fell into the following categories as seen in figure 4.3 below.

**Figure 4.3** Delayed Discharges Figures for Year End March 2023.

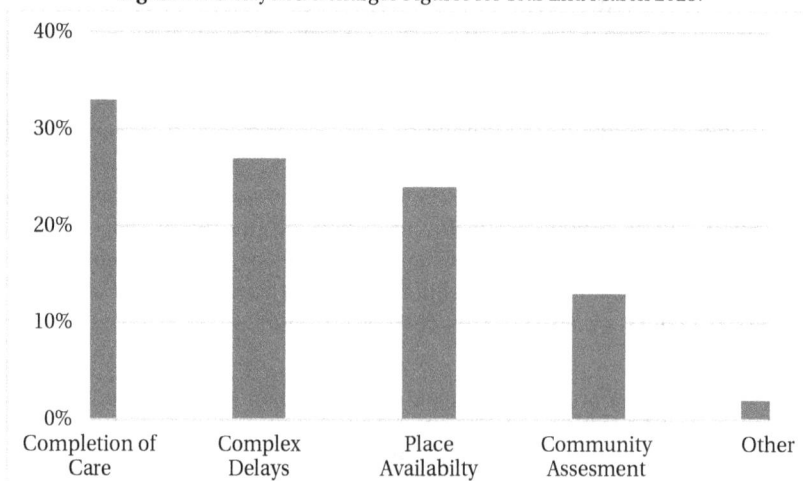

Data from: Public Health Scotland (2023) *Delayed discharges in NHS Scotland, annual: Annual summary of occupied beds and census figures, data to March 2023. Edinburgh*: A National Statistics publication for Scotland. Available at: https://publichealthscotland.scot/publications/delayed-discharges-in-nhsscotland-annual/delayed-discharges-in-nhsscotland-annual-annual-summary-of-occupied-bed-days-and-census-figures-data-to-march-2023/. Accessed: 10th October 2023.

Sam spoke of the problems of having delayed discharge of patients on their ward:

> We have one wee man that is in, and he is dead confused, now we keep telling the doctors that he is confused, we see him all the time…. but they say he has capacity. He wants to go back to his own home, but he is not going to be safe…. They (the family) need to apply for guardianship, but that's another thing, it could take over a year. So, that wee man is going to be with us for…. until he dies. (Sam, 2023).

One reason Sam gave, as to why patients were experiencing delayed discharge, was for "house cleaning". In this situation, the patient is no longer a medical problem but a social one. For those with complex needs, a home assessment will be carried out before discharge. If the home assessment team, comprising of a physiotherapist, an occupational therapist and a social worker, deem the house to be unsafe, due to cleanliness, a house clean will be organised. According to Sam, this could include new carpets, bedding etc. This is all charged to the NHS Scotland. I am unsure if this just occurs in Scotland or if it is a UK-wide policy. The house cleaning can take months before it is completed due to staff shortages within social care.

Research by Ben-Harush et al. (2017) investigated ageism amongst medical and social care staff, identifying three themes:

- Perceived difficulties in working with the elderly and their families
- The elderly as an invisible group, leading to a bias of communication and inappropriate care
- Problems resulted in a "manifestation of ageism". (Ben-Harush et al. 2017, p. 39)

The researchers questioned why ageism exists within the medical profession. Do we all exhibit ageism as a defence against our ageing and declining health? Do we see frailty in others as a reminder of our mortality? Whatever the reasons, the result of ageism within the medical profession remains the same it "affects the quality of treatment and the services that older adults receive" (Ben-Harush et al. 2017, p. 40). The bias of ageism will be examined in the following two sections concerning poor communication and the placing of DNR orders on the elderly.

### Do Not Resuscitate Orders (DNR)

When I took a call from the IRH at 3.30 am on 30th March 2020, I was somewhat unprepared for the conversation that followed with an A&E consultant doctor. I was told that my dad had been admitted to A&E with COVID-19 and that my dad had authorised me to make any decisions regarding his end-of-life care. I was then asked if I would place a DNR order on him. I agreed immediately. As an ex-nurse, I recognised just how traumatic resuscitation was, especially for the elderly. I knew that coronary pulmonary resuscitation (CPR) carried a risk of "bruising, broken ribs and punctured lungs" (Bows and Herring, 2022, p. 61). I did not want that for my dad. I was also aware of just how small the success rate was with around only 10 – 20% of people having a positive outcome. (Bows and Herring, 2022). Importantly, this was a decision I made in the best interests of my dad, this is not, and should not be, a universal decision for all elderly people.

Following the pandemic, there have been a lot of stories in the UK media about the perceived excessive use of DNR orders, placed on the elderly and those with diminished intellectual capacity during the pandemic.[11] Concerns were raised that the orders were being placed on people simply because they inhabited the aforementioned two demographics and that decisions were being made on the group, not the individual person. DNR orders are necessary to allow those who are terminally ill the right to die with dignity. They are a necessary part of a doctor's arsenal for good and appropriate patient care. Yet, could it be, as Coleman argues, that doctors who place DNR orders without the consent of the patient simply because of their age perform "a form of eugenics" (2022, p. 23).

Following a ruling in 2014, the British Court of Appeal deemed that it was a breach of human rights not to consult a patient before placing a DNR order on them. This followed a judicial review on a case where a woman died after having two DNR orders placed on her without her, or her family's consent or knowledge:

> Lawyers Leigh Day, on behalf of the Tracey family, argued that the imposition of a DNACPR order on a patient with capacity, without first informing them or giving them any opportunity to express their views was a breach under Article 8 of the Human Rights Act, which provides that: "Everyone has the right to respect for their private and family life". (Leigh Day, 2014).

Although changes were put in place to ensure proper practice over DNR orders, COVID-19 saw those fall by the wayside, thwarted by the many challenges the pandemic brought.

---

[11] At the time of writing this book the UK is holding a public enquiry into the UK government's handling of the pandemic. This also involves examining the individual devolved administrations and is looking at, amongst other issues, the use of DNR orders.

My own experience with my dad's initial admission, and the conversation with the consultant, resonated with Tomkow et al. (2022) research findings:

- Almost half of all DNR orders were made in A&E departments.
- Almost all conversations with relatives took place over the telephone.
- Orders were placed without consulting the patient.
- Orders were placed on groups of people with no individuality.

The first two outcomes are not that surprising. The rapid deterioration of a patient with COVID-19, especially during the first wave, meant that priority was placed on stabilising the patient. There was no time to consider making an end-of-life care plan. With the country on lockdown, all conversations with families regarding DNR orders had to take place over the telephone, there were no face-to-face consultations. The final two findings are concerning. Having read this research, I have had to reflect on my own experience. As mentioned, I was told my dad wanted me to make the decision, I did so without a second thought as these were his wishes, and he trusted my judgement. Yet after I had spoken to the doctor, she had a nurse call me on my dad's mobile to enable me to *say my goodbyes*. My dad was very breathless and understandably distressed, but he was, and remained until his death, very lucid. I am now left with doubts that he had been consulted, and that he had wanted me to make the decision. I fear that the doctor asked me because they knew I was an ex-nurse and had probably seen CPR being performed. As a result, I would be more likely to have the order put in place than perhaps my dad would. Cherniak looked at research into DNR orders placed on elderly patients in both the US and UK and found that "several studies of 100 – 200 patients each noted a majority favouring CPR…. Despite these findings, there is evidence that while many elderly favour resuscitation, they die with DNR orders in place." (2002, p. 303). I wonder if they had assessed the need for an order simply because of his elderly status, as my dad remained hopeful of a full recovery until just before his death. Was there an element of ageism? Did the doctor *bypass* my dad to gain a more favourable response from me?

I was also left with a feeling of disquiet when I read Bows and Herring's research findings. They looked at the concerns raised over the impression that DNR orders were placed, as a matter of routine, on the elderly. Interestingly, following an analysis of 126,545 patients with a DNA order in place, they found that although the number of DNR orders increased during the first wave, there was not a significant increase within the elderly group. The increase was to be found within the middle-aged group. What they also discovered, however, was "that Black Caribbean patients were over-represented in the sample analysed"

(2022, p. 80).[12] This is something that requires more research. They also reported that despite it being a breach of human rights, over a fifth of patients, and their families, in the sample, were not consulted before the DNR order was placed on their notes.

Roseanne was asked on more than one occasion to place a DNR order on her mum, but she refused. The first time she was asked correlated with both my own experience and with research findings (Bows and Herring, 2022; Tomkow et al., 2023) in that the request was unexpected and by telephone:

> The doctor came on the phone – 'your mother's deteriorated a wee bit. We don't have a DNR in place. We need this.' I said I wasn't signing it, so they asked me to come over to the hospital. Oh, I thought, now they want me involved. So, I went in; the doctor says 'come on let's chat about this. Your mother's 76, she lives alone, she's got two home helps, why won't you put a DNR in place?' (Roseanne, 2022).

What stands out from Roseanne's transcript is that at no point does she mention that she has given any information about what CPR involves, the risks, and the success rate. It also appears, from the transcript, that she was not given any opportunity to ask questions. When she refused again to authorise the order, she was told that the hospital would take it out of her hands and place the order anyway. This overruling of the family has been noted in other research papers (Tomkow et al., 2023).

Although Roseanne and her family were initially separated from their mum due to the national lockdown, when she refused to agree to the order over the telephone, they asked her to come to the ward. Tomkow et al. analysed the responses to the request compared to the amount of information known or given. They found that those who had or received good information on CPR had a more positive experience with the way the situation was handled, and their family member cared for. They noted that many of those who had little knowledge "reported learning about the subject from television medical dramas" (2023, p. 4). Raising the question of a DNR order brings to the fore many emotions for the family, feelings of guilt and anger over the burden of responsibility. Others, in Tomkow et al.'s research, spoke of anger towards the hospital staff and a feeling that the hospital no longer wanted to care for their relative, something Roseanne can attest to "I know she wasn't getting that care, and that's the biggest thing for me." Yet, as Ben-Harush et al. point out, "avoidance

---

[12] I felt uneasy as a close friend's brother had died, in April 2020, during the first wave of the pandemic. He was only 50 years old and belonged to the Black Caribbean demographic. I asked my friend about an DNR order, but she told me that during the two weeks he was in hospital he had been administered CPR on three separate occasions.

of invasive medical treatment can be perceived as compassionate care" (2017, p. 40). Invasive treatment can be painful, frightening and, ultimately, futile. Roseanne and I made different decisions for our parents when it came to placing a DNR order, we both acted in their best interests. We had the privilege of knowing the individual, the medical staff only knew them as an elderly patient.

### Poor communication

In 2022 Ramya Sampath looked at the shift which positioned iatrogenic disease as negligent behaviour. One major concern was the lack of communication with the patient. They argued that, by removing the patient's autonomy, not only was the patient exposed to iatrogenic disease, but this became a negligent act carried out by the hospital staff. Lack of communication is a prime example of the problems highlighted by Pilnick (2023) over PCC and the presence of deontic authority. With the elderly patient not falling into the perceived 'ideal' patient "the empowerment promised by PCC isn't easily achieved" (Pilnick, 2023, p. 3). Sampath's research paper examined poor communication and an overriding of patients' wishes when it came to family involvement in their care. I was immediately reminded of Tracy's dad's distress when his stepdaughter visited. Even though Tracy had invited her stepsister to the hospital where their dad was admitted, there had been no contact between them for many years. When their dad saw his stepdaughter, he became deeply distressed, to the point where medical staff had to administer a sedative. Consequently, the family had to request that the stepsister leave the hospital. At this point, a memo was placed on John's notes that this member of the family was to be given no information about their dad, and all communication was to be directed to Tracy. The following day, the charge nurse took a call from the stepdaughter and told her to come to the hospital straight away as her dad had deteriorated. His answer, when Tracy challenged him on this, was that her stepsister had a right to know that her dad was critically ill. Tracy later complained about the charge nurse to the hospital, but that day, she had reprimanded him herself:

> [y]ou are working in a coronary care ward where the patient's rights should come first, not the.... I mean, you don't even know if that is his real daughter that's phoned, and you've just said, "aye come in!" (Tracy, 2022).

Nothing came of her formal complaint. Yet Sampath's findings are relevant in this case "determining iatrogenic harm must depend on whether a patient's wishes for familial involvement are honored" (2022, p. 737). If the stepdaughter had gained access to John's room the potential for iatrogenesis was high. There can be an argument for the involvement of all family members during end-of-life care. It may be viewed as callous or cruel to exclude a particular family member from saying their goodbyes or making their piece with a dying relative. However, all that the medical staff can do is attempt to mediate with the separate factions, because when all is said and done, the patient's wishes are paramount. Iatrogenic harm must be prevented "during their most vulnerable periods of life" (Sampath, 2022, p. 738). The ward had written down John's wishes so that there could be no ambiguity over the issue of his stepdaughter's involvement during his hospital admission. To ignore a written directive is negligent behaviour.

The bias that can be shown against elderly patients can take many forms. It can range from not speaking directly to the elderly patient during consultations, to being less respectful and pessimistic when discussing treatments and outcomes. It can even go as far as not recommending invasive cancer treatments, something that, perhaps, can be argued is treating the patient with compassion. What was of interest were the findings of Ben-Harush et al. when it came to nurses' behaviour, a group that was also less optimistic when it came to outcomes over rehabilitation. It was noted, when observing a group of Scottish nurses, that they "used shallow language and shouted, without any humour and without even addressing the patients by name" (2017, p. 40). Yet, the UK is not alone in having problems within its healthcare sector. Ellis and Standing pointed out that "healthcare failures are a worldwide problem… many of the failures and complaints relate not to care per se, but more often to how care is delivered, poor communication and lack of information giving." (2023, p. 8). One comment I received on TikTok confirmed this statement:

> The content creator wrote about having similar issues in Canada. In their opinion nothing had improved in senior healthcare for more than a decade. (A, TikTok, 2022).

Today, many adult children find themselves advocating for their parents when it comes to navigating medical care. Research into ageism noted that medical staff are inadequately trained and, therefore, ill-prepared when it comes to working with the elderly and their families. As a result, they have perceived difficulties in working collaboratively with them (Ben-Harush et al. 2017). A major problem is one of communication with "[t]he use of condescending and infantilizing language" (Ben-Harush et al. 2017, p. 46) when talking to the elderly patient being noted. Yet, the engagement of both the elderly patient and their families is "an ethical imperative that embraces the principles of inclusivity, mutual respect and co-design" (Holroyd-Leduc et al. 2016, p. 2). Following the principles of PCC, enabling autonomy through engagement improves not only the experiences of the patient at the time of the interaction but can also lead to better health outcomes (Holroyd-Leduc et al. 2016). It is alarming that many health professionals ignore the elderly patient when deciding on a care plan, by either discussing the situation with family members or simply making the decision themselves with no consultation (Ben-Harush et al. 2017).

Holroyd-Leduc et al.'s Canadian research examined giving the elderly a voice when it came to their health care. Their research examined frail elderly adults who were cared for by the informal family caregiving network. The emphasis was on PCC, and engagement with the elderly adult but also brought to the fore family-centred care (FPC), noting that "in any setting, family caregivers play an important role in engaging and empowering older adults living with family" (2016, p. 2). To ensure a good level of care, the family and medical practitioners must come together to ensure that the elderly patient's autonomy is preserved. Sam's transcript gives an example of good communication with the family. They overheard a patient complaining to her daughter that the nurses were not following the rehabilitation plan the physiotherapists had set out for her:

> I heard her say "the physios told me I had to walk with my stick [under supervision] but the nurses just aren't interested". I went over and explained that I knew her mum was supposed to get up and walk with one of the nurses, but we were just so short staffed. I explained that Monday – Friday the physios came in and took her for a walk and that at other times she had her zimmer and been walking up and down the ward. Once I explained that it wasn't like she wasn't doing any walking the daughter understood, but you still feel bad, you feel so bad, because you can't deal with it, you can't do it. (Sam, 2023).

The research I carried out for this chapter left me with more questions than answers when it came to the care our parents received at the QEUH. The reasons behind the increased use of DNR orders and midazolam will never be known. It was a constant battle not to be drawn down the *rabbit hole* of conspiracy theories. Yet one MSP's view could not be ignored. Angus Robertson's views on the increased deaths of the elderly at the beginning of the pandemic were put to print in an article titled "The Momentum is With Us" for *The National* Newspaper. Mr Robertson wrote:

> [s]ince 2014, opinions have clearly not been static, and polls have shown a gradual rise in support for independence…. This could be in significant part because of the underlying change in the electorate, with roughly 55,000 predominantly Yes supporting 16-year-olds joining the electorate and 55,000 predominantly No supporting older voters passing away every year…. Since 2014, this has added around 330,000 voters to the electorate, with a likely net gain of over 100,000 for independence. (Robertson, quoted in Gordon, 2020).

Every cloud seemingly does have a silver lining.

One way in which we can look to improve the care given to the elderly is by having geriatric care specialists. This area of care would see geriatricians "managing the complex needs of frail and elderly patients by working alongside a growing number of superspecialists" (McKee et al. 2021). With the problems of chronic staff shortages, it is difficult to see just how this can be achieved. As was discussed in Chapter Three, these shortages have contributed to falling morale within the NHS and nurses are now suffering from both physical and psychological burnout. To compound the problem budget cuts have seen health boards put a halt on nurse recruitment whilst staff retention remains a worry.

## Chapter Five

# The Queen Elizabeth University Hospital: The Death Star

## Yvonne Bennett

This chapter will discuss the QEUH and the problems that have plagued it since its opening in 2015. We will consider findings from the public enquiry alongside testimony from staff members, patients, and their relatives. This hospital was heralded as the Scottish government's flagship project and is known locally as The Death Star. It initially gained its moniker because its imposing 14-storey star-shaped design reminded people of the gargantuan space station, The Death Star, in the Star Wars franchise. However, for the participants in this study, and all those who contacted me via TikTok with their stories, it has taken on a more ominous meaning, as a place of death as opposed to healing. Sadly, for Roseanne, who lives close by, it is a daily visual reminder of the trauma she experienced over her mum's care and subsequent death. My first visit to the QEUH occurred at 1.30 am on Thursday, 11th August 2022, as I waited outside A&E for my mum to arrive by ambulance. What struck me most was the size of the building, and I quickly became aware of complications that occur due to the sheer dimension of the building. It took me 15 minutes to find my way to A&E from the car park. As I waited in the hospital, and the hours passed by, I became aware of more and more problems; talking to staff, experiencing my difficulties as a visitor, and noting how the hospital design impacted patient care.

### Patient Concerns

I was drawn to the doctoral thesis by Seyed Ashrafi, where, on a visit to a hospital, they observed that the hospital environment was incapable of meeting the needs of the patients and their families when it came to basic non-medical necessities such as comfort and dignity. The blame was not caused by medical practitioners' negligence but because "designers mostly focused on what was necessary for the treatment process" (2017, p. 13). This preoccupation rendered hospitals as simply a place of treatment and did not take into consideration the wider non-medical requirements of people. Not all who visit a hospital are ill. This lack of appropriate response to the overall hospital population's needs was apparent when my mum was transferred to an orthopaedic ward on the tenth floor of the hospital. As can be seen in image 2.4, Chapter Two, the QEUH is built with four wings stemming from a central atrium. Each wing has access to the floors via two lift blocks, one used for patient transfer, and the other for staff and visitors. The issues concern all of the lift blocks and are caused by their design, as the lifts only travel to pre-selected floors. To call the lift you must press the number of the floor you require; a display then tells you whether you have been allocated lift A, B, or C. If another lift arrives before the one you have been allotted, you cannot use it as there are no *call floor* buttons inside the lift. It will only stop at pre-designated floors. If your lift arrives and it is full, you must start the process over. I spent a lot of time waiting for a lift. I must also add that due to frustration, at the length of time spent waiting, people would cram into the lifts at a time when social distancing was still in place. I wondered how much time staff wasted at break time, waiting for lifts to take them down to the café areas, and how much time was lost getting staff, such as physiotherapists or pharmacists, to and from different wards during their working hours. One QEUH worker was quoted in the Scottish media as saying they had spent "the majority of my time in the lift since the building opened, as have a lot of people" (Parry, 2015). When the QEUH first opened, hospital management enlisted volunteers to explain to people the correct way in which to operate the lifts. Although that service has now been stopped, I learned during this research that many people, especially the elderly, still have problems when it comes to using the lifts correctly (Tracy, 2022; Sam, 2023). This specific lift problem was not confined to the visitor and staff lifts but also concerned the patient transfer lifts, or, as they are known by hospital staff, core lifts. Jordan spoke of one experience when transferring a patient. As the patient was medically unstable, a nurse escort was with them:

> [w]e put in that we wanted the ground floor and we waited and waited and waited. The nurse said 'this is ridiculous' and we waited and waited and eventually a porter arrived. Luckily, he had a pass that he scanned which allowed the lift to come straight away. (Jordan, 2022).

A second area of concern is the design of the wards. The wards have 100% single occupancy rooms with ensuite facilities; the rooms are large and are set out in a semi-circular design with four wards on each floor. There is a nursing station situated about halfway around the ward and, from here, nurses have a clear line of visibility to about three or four rooms.[1] This, especially where there is a high percentage of elderly patients, causes problems. Many of the elderly

---

[1] I must point out that I am writing this section from memory and this number may not be accurate. I cannot remember how many rooms were on each ward and have been unable to find this out.

patients in my mum's ward were categorised as a *fall risk*.[2] To ensure their safety, these patients were sat in the doorways of their rooms with a nurse/ auxiliary sitting opposite them. There were three immediate problems that I could envisage from this practice:

- Deduction of a staff member from the ward routine
- Loss of dignity
- Isolation

As has been noted in Chapter Two, the QEUH suffers from chronic staff shortages. Placing one staff member on *watch duty* excludes that person from undertaking daily ward duty tasks such as attending to the personal hygiene needs of the patients, exacerbating staff shortages. Any ward using such a practice is short-staffed from the outset. The second problem is the loss of dignity. Once again, I was minded of Ashrafi's work:

> designers have a responsibility to plan hospitals in such a way as to help ensure that patient's rights can be suitably addressed... Accordingly, designers should be expected to provide environments that are responsive to the dignity and rights of patients. (2017, p. 95).

Dignity is defined by Lothian and Philp as "an individual maintaining self-respect and being valued by others" (2001, p. 668); there can be no dignity when one is sat in a doorway viewed by all who pass by, be they staff or visitors. Ashrafi maintained that dignity must be given optimum consideration when hospitals were being designed, noting they "found the concept of dignity instrumental in giving an idea to designers about the ethical requirements of people in hospitals" (2017, p. 14). However, different hospital designers may have different solutions when it comes to safeguarding patient dignity. Ashrafi argued that the use of single rooms aided in the preservation of dignity as it afforded the patient and their visitors privacy. That single rooms enhance both dignity and privacy when it comes to personal care is not disputed (Singh and Okeke, 2016). On a personal note, if I were to have the misfortune to require hospital care, I would want to have a single occupancy room, but my needs were so different from those of my mum. This emphasises the problem of not taking into account the divergent needs of the elderly and, therefore placing them in the path of iatrogenic harm.

There are many benefits to be had for single occupancy rooms, not least, improved infection control. However, single occupancy rooms or some elderly

---

[2] I had questioned the nursing staff about the patients sitting in doorways being observed by a member of the nursing team and I was informed that these patients had been categorised as a fall risk.

are akin to solitary confinement highlighting the second problem, that of isolation. Anderson et al. investigated infection control in nursing homes during the pandemic. They proposed that "a balance must be struck among social engagement, communal activities and infection control" (2020, p. 1522). They acknowledged the challenges faced by staff working in the care of the elderly facility. There is a daily struggle trying to strike a balance between infection control and the mental health consequences of social isolation. Despite being sat partially in the corridor, as the rooms in the QEUH are spacious, the doorways have a large area between them, therefore the patients are unable to communicate properly with each other, as one ex-nurse commented:

> The QEUH is not suitable for the elderly, they are confined alone in their single rooms and far from the nurses' station. We cannot see them, and this makes it so unsafe. (TikTok respondent, 2022).

Singh and Okeke also emphasised the problems of loneliness and social isolation, commenting that "new hospitals need to be designed to meet the needs of old and frailer populations and a generalised *one size fits all* guideline should not be applied" (2016, p. 8). Jordan mentioned their aunt finding it difficult in the single rooms as she is registered blind with core morbidities that necessitate hospital admissions. Prior to the QEUH she would be admitted to the Western Infirmary and would be in an old Nightingale ward.[3]

> [i]t was ideal because everybody (staff and patients) was in the same area. My auntie might need a bit of help…. And if there wasn't a nurse to help, she would always have made a pal, and they would help each other out. (Jordan, 2022).

This is consistent with research findings, which noted that the old style multi bedded wards were "often in the line of vision of staff, and there is an added benefit of increased surveillance by other patients and relatives" (Singh and Okeke, 2016, p. 2).

Just as there should be doctors and nurses who specialise in the care of the elderly, (Lothian and Philps, 2001; McKee et al., 2021), Permpongkosol suggested that one way in which to prevent iatrogenic harm in the elderly is to "create wards specifically for the elderly" (2011, p. 80). Yet, this does not appear to be taken into consideration when new hospitals are being designed and built. Singh and Okeke looked at the increased number of elderly in-patient falls in the Ysbyty Ystrad Fawr (YYF) hospital in Wales. The YYF is a newly built hospital and, like the QEUH, has been built with 100% single occupancy rooms. The YYF

---

[3] The Nightingale wards were named after Florence Nightingale and were large single gender wards with beds down on either side against the wall. There were usually about 30 patients in a ward with the nurses' station in the centre.

opened in 2011, replacing two older hospitals, and has three specialist care of the elderly wards (Singh and Okeke, 2016). Shortly after opening, the YYF's patient safety team raised concerns about the increased number of in-patient falls. Despite no changes in demographic or bed numbers between the previous two hospitals and the YYF, the patient safety team noted "an IF (in-patient fall) rate almost 2.5 times higher as compared to the two previous hospitals" (Singh and Okeke, 2016, p. 1). Their research also highlighted the aforementioned problems of isolation and less supervision by staff as patients are less visible from the nursing station. Not only are nurses not able to observe a patient in their room but due to the size of the wards, there is an increase in time getting to a room to respond to a call bell. Based on their findings, Singh and Okeke recommended that other health authorities follow YYF's lead in giving all nurses regular fall risk training. This is in accordance with NICE's framework on the prevention of elderly in-patient falls.[4] At the time of Singh and Okeke's research the YYF had reported "a reduction of 34% in a high risk 100% single room environment" (2016, p. 8) following extensive nurse training in elderly fall risk. However, the rate remains higher in the YYF than in the previous two hospitals combined.

To address the problem of in-patient falls at QEUH, one staff member suggested that all rooms be equipped with cameras. This does bring into question the right of the patient to privacy. It is, of course, recognised that privacy is a basic human right and one that must be respected by all health professionals. To do otherwise could have a detrimental impact on the patient's physical and mental well-being. Nonetheless, does the placing of cameras in a room have a greater impact on privacy than sitting patients in doorways? One way that was suggested to overcome the issue of privacy was to obtain patient consent for the camera to be on when the patient was occupying the room. If the patient refused, the camera would be switched off. There are already 450 surveillance cameras in situ in heavily trafficked areas both inside and outside the main QEUH hospital building (North Tec, 2023).[5] These cameras are operated for the safety of all who work and use the hospital. The obvious argument is that cameras installed in rooms are necessary to ensure the safety of those deemed a fall risk. Patient safety is being compromised when a solution is available. This

---

[4] NICE is the National Institute for Health and Care Excellence is a UK government organisation which provides evidence bases guidance for health care professionals. Their guidance on fall prevention for the elderly is available at: https://www.nice.org.uk/guidance/cg161

[5] Information from North Tec, the company who installed and maintain the security systems at the QEUH. Available from: https://north.tech/case-studies/queen-elizabeth-university-hospital/

is an example of a disregard for the elderly and their specific needs at a time when the number of elderly in Scotland is increasing.

Ashrafi's work and observations show just how much the environment can affect the daily lives of all who inhabit the hospital setting, be they patients, visitors, or staff. They put forward that the goal of a hospital is to provide quality care for people when they are ill, vulnerable, and dependent. Ashrafi proposes that "[t]his goal can be achieved if hospital designers focus on two main missions. Firstly, to prevent a person's condition from deteriorating and, secondly, to attempt to make it better" (2017, p. 16). Based on these findings, a hospital must be designed in such a way that it optimises an individual's personal abilities. If this goal is to be met, then hospital architectures must have as the foundation of their design the following ethical principles:

- Design for vulnerability
- Design for healing
- Design for reverence (Ashrafi, 2017, p. 16).

Although one could argue that by the use of single rooms, the QEUH has these three principles within its framework. However, it has taken all patients as a homogenous group and has not looked specifically at the elderly, especially those with dementia. In doing so, the designers of the QEUH have placed the elderly at risk of iatrogenic harm, both physically, through falls and mentally through social isolation.

According to its patient charter, merely healing people is not the only goal of the NHS; it is also concerned about the quality of care and the condition of the people who use its services alongside its staff. The physical environment of hospitals must be taken into consideration when meeting this goal (Department of Health, 2015). When people are in crisis, they are at their most vulnerable. It is essential that they receive the care and support they need as quickly as possible, in a place they can feel safe, and, that they are supported by people who understand their needs (Care Quality Commission Act (2014)).[6] On the basis of their findings, Anderson et al. call to our attention the "urgent need to examine these [care facility] design models" (2020, p. 1519). By taking into account the specific health and social care needs of the elderly, designers can utilise approaches that improve quality of life whilst not compromising infection control or safety.

The treatment of the patient's relatives and visitors at such a stressful time was also called into question. Tracy and Jamie-Lee spoke of their own family needs being disregarded, an issue that was highlighted by Ashrafi. The dignity

---

[6] The Care Quality Commission Act (2014) can be accessed at www.cqc.org.uk.

of the patient's family must also be considered, especially at a time when that family member may not be taking into account their own needs. Ashrafi pointed out that if there were no facilities in the room for the family member to rest or if they were not being offered food or drinks, then they "may prefer to stay near to their hospitalised family member and endure the tiredness or hunger rather than going outside of the hospital premises to find something to eat, or somewhere to rest." (2017, p. 118).

> [t]hey never even gave us a comfortable chair…. and we were left for two days. Never even gave us a blanket or anything…. I was there for ten hours, and they didn't even offer me anything to drink. (Tracy, 2022).

Despite the rooms being spacious Tracy and her dad's former partner were not offered the use of a recliner chair, a blanket, or anything to eat or drink. I could not find a clause in NHS Scotland's charter regarding food and care for patients' visitors but NHS England's national standard for healthcare food and drink states in section 3.4:

> [o]rganisations must provide access to suitable food and drink out of hours (based on the above nutrition standards). What this means in practice: This standard ensures all staff and visitors are given equal opportunity to access food and drink that supports their nutrition and hydration needs 24/7 including drinking water.[7]

The QEUH has vending machines offering food and drinks on every floor.[8] There are also food outlets in the atrium on the ground floor. However, if, like Tracy, you have left home in an emergency without sufficient money to buy food or drink, then the ward staff must offer some refreshments. Neglecting Tracy's own needs placed her in substantial iatrogenic harm through dehydration and falling blood sugar.

It is not only the elderly who are at risk of iatrogenic harm due to the single rooms and the inability of patient observation to be carried out. Both Sam and Jordan spoke of in-patient suicides in the QEUH:

> I don't know if you've heard – there's numerous people that have committed suicide in the wards. (Jordan, 2022).

---

[7] NHS England's National Standards for healthcare food and drink can be accessed at: https://www.england.nhs.uk/publication/national-standards-for-healthcare-food-and-drink/

[8] When my mum was admitted the vending machine on her floor was not working. The food outlets were also, in my opinion expensive, especially if you were there unable to go home for any considerable period of time.

That morning, I came in and the girls (nurses) were all talking about something that had happened the night before. It was a young guy, obviously, I think there is a big investigation going on. So, I think the young guy, I don't know if he had poor mobility or something, but they had found him dead in the shower. The night before. They just found him dead in lying the shower. They were talking about how long he had been lying there and they didn't know how long he had been lying there or anything, because he was independent, that was the thing. (Sam, 2023).

NHS Scotland has witnessed 50 suicides since 2015, with 20 of these being under the NHSGGC health board jurisdiction. It appears that, despite these tragic deaths, the QEUH was not only not suicide proofed but "has been built with ligature points – places where a noose can be hung – against the recommendation of its own ruling board" (Leask 2016). Yet again, the problem of being unable to observe patients has resulted in iatrogenic harm. The failure to ensure that a new hospital is built in such a manner as to make suicides impossible can be classed as negligent. The architects that designed the QEUH appear to have only implemented one of Asfari's design principles, that is the principle of reverence. The building does indeed bring a sense of awe but in all other aspects, appears unfit for purpose.

### Timeline of problems at QEUH

**2015**

- A premature baby dies of a bacterial infection. Five other babies in the unit tested positive for the infection.

- A terminally ill man waits for over eight hours to be seen at A&E.

**2016**

- A child within ward 2A was identified as having a bloodstream infection (BSI) as a result of Cupriavidus pauculus, a waterborne bacterium.

- Ten cases are recorded of children contracting fungal infections whilst in-patients at QEUH.

**2017**

- A child dies after her Hickman line is contaminated by a bacterial infection during a stem cell transplant. She was one of 84 children who were exposed to and later infected with a rare bacterium who were all there to receive treatment for blood disease, cancer, or related conditions.

- A further 26 cases of a fungal infection are recorded. These affect 14 children.
- Three patients were found to have died with Stenotrophomonas maltophilia, a waterborne bacterium, in their bloodstream.
- The hospital building was found to have cladding similar to what was used to construct the Grenfell Tower.[9]

**2018**

- Three more children are treated for waterborne infections.
- 23 children in cancer wards 2A and 2B were found to have contracted bloodstream infections from contaminated taps, wash basins and drains.
- Children's wards 2A and 2B are closed and the water supply is shut down to allow for chlorine dousing to treat the bacterial contamination.

**2019**

- Two patients died from a bacterial infection caused by pigeon droppings. One was a ten-year-old boy receiving cancer treatment.
- An investigation has begun into the death of a three-year-old boy.

**2020**

- Andrew Slorance, a Scottish Government communication expert, dies after contracting a fungal infection caused by mould. The cause of death is not noted on his death certificate.

**2021**

- Mr Slorance's widow complains of a cover-up over her husband's death.
- The final inquiry report notes that since 2015 "84 children and young people between them experienced 118 episodes of infection. At least 33 of these episodes probably related to the hospital environment, and two children and young people had died due to their infection." (Scottish Labour, 2021).

---

[9] Grenfell Tower was a 23-story tower block in London. At 1 am on the 14th of June 2017, a fire broke out in a fourth-floor apartment kitchen. The blaze quickly spread up the outside of the tower block on all four sides due to its highly flammable cladding. Within two hours all of the upper floors were alight and 72 people lost their lives.

**2022**

- Work is underway to remove and replace some of the wall panels within the atrium. It is predicted that the work will take around five years for £33million.

- Ambulances are waiting in queues for up to two hours before dropping patients off at A&E.

**2023**

- Confirmation that Raac has been found in older buildings on the QEUH campus.

- A glass panel fell to the ground. No injuries were reported.

- NHSGGC is named as a suspect in a corporate homicide investigation into the deaths of four patients: a ten-year-old girl, a ten-year-old boy, a three-year-old boy and a 75-year-old-woman.

### Staff Concerns

Further problems were brought to my attention when I was in the A&E department waiting for my mum to be assessed. I started chatting to a member of staff and they spoke of the problems they experienced due to the size of the hospital and the combining of five major hospitals onto one site. They spoke of no longer knowing who they were working with, of there being a sense of a team or camaraderie. This member of staff also spoke of the differences in working in a small department of perhaps 20 people compared to now working with over 250. A concern was knowing the strengths and weaknesses of the staff they were working with. They explained to me that as a senior member of staff, they needed to know who was proficient at tasks and required zero or minimal supervision as opposed to those who were recently qualified. Professional concerns aside, they also lamented the loss of work friendships. The following is my side of the conversation during the interview with Sam:

> [t]hey told me that you don't see the same person twice so you can't build up a rapport or you can't have a laugh or a joke or ask, 'how is so and so?' They didn't know when someone has left or not. They told me that they have got every piece of shiny equipment in that hospital (QEUH) that you could wish for, they just don't have the people to work it. They also told me of recently bumping into a colleague they hadn't seen in a while and asked the colleague how she was. They were shocked to be told that she was just returning from maternity leave. This member of staff explained that they hadn't even known the colleague was

pregnant never mind knowing she had a baby and had been off for months.

My conversation with this staff member finished when I left to take a phone call from my brother, and as I headed out, they called after me, "wait until you hear about the difficulties the domestic staff have". I did not have long to wait.

The housekeeping/domestic staff have many problems with the cleaning of such a large building. Each ward/department has its own housekeeping team, but when a patient is discharged, a designated team is sent to the ward to clean and sanitise the room.[10] When my mum arrived at the ward, the room she was to occupy hadn't been cleaned; we had to wait in the corridor for around 30 minutes until the designated housekeeping staff arrived. They were extremely apologetic, but, like everyone else, they had had a long wait for a lift. I must apologise for uttering the cliché phrase *in my day*, but there is no way around it. I began nursing in January 1981 when I was 17 ½ years old, I had spent the previous six months working in a care home. Throughout my 12 years in the profession, when a patient was discharged, it was all nursing staff: auxiliaries, students and RGNs who cleaned the room or bay prior to a new admission. This included stripping and cleaning the bed and cleaning the locker with disinfectant before remaking the bed with clean linen, it would take around 15 minutes to do. Now, a designated team had to be called, and time was lost waiting for them to arrive; it also took longer to clean the room, and the ensuite as both were quite large. The housekeeping staff were rushed as they had more rooms to clean in other wards before admissions. The lack of cleanliness was noted by Tracy, Jamie-Lee and Roseanne:

> **Tracy**: one of the patients opposite my dad passed away. They took the bed out of the room, sprayed the bed, sprayed something into the room, didnae wipe handles or anything, didnae wipe anything and just put the bed back in. Honestly it was like a conveyor belt. That room should have been…
>
> **Jamie-Lee**: scrubbed…
>
> **Tracy**: sanitised…
>
> **Jamie-Lee**: especially if someone has just passed away in there, it's not just normal germs…
>
> **Tracy**: she just came in, sprayed, like, a spray, didnae even shut the room door…

---

[10] I spoke to a nurse friend who works at another Glasgow hospital, and they informed me that the nursing staff clean the bed area/room when a patient is discharged. They do not have a designated domestic team.

> **Jamie-Lee**: it was as if she could nae be really bothered by it all, the workload is…
>
> **Tracy**: the mattress, it was in the corridor, it was sprayed in the corridor and then put it back in. Did nae wash the wee unit, did nae wash the handles of the doors, the toilet, nothing.
>
> **Tracy**: at four o'clock in the morning a domestic came in dropped this *bomb* thing in the sink, in my dad's room, and said 'I. should have done that hours ago. 'I mean at four o'clock in the morning when we are trying to sleep….

Roseanne also spoke of her mum's room not being clean and the shock of finding the previous occupant's possessions and medication in the bedside locker. One benefit of single rooms is it aids in the prevention of the spread of infection. However, this can only happen if basic hygiene rules are being followed.

Sam and Jordan also raised concerns over the size of the hospital, with both noting that on several occasions, they had wandered around the QEUH staff-only areas and no one had questioned them. In a smaller unit, people know who staff members are and can challenge those they do not recognise; this is a large security risk. Both also highlighted the lack of camaraderie between different departments, with nurses in A&E no longer knowing the paramedics or the physiotherapists:

> [y]ou used to know all you're A&E nurses and they knew all their ambulance drivers…. We used to have nights out with the A&E staff. That doesn't happen here [QEUH]. It used to, years ago but that changed. You can go and never see the same face again. (Jordan, 2022).

Research into workplace environments highlights the importance of knowing your colleagues as it promotes an atmosphere that is conducive to increased productivity. Knowing your colleagues helps to foster a workplace environment that "caters to individual needs" (Indeed, 2023). Within an organisation such as the NHS, where different health professionals are coming together to meet the needs of patients, one should take into consideration Frans Johansson's central theme from his 2004 book *The Medici Effect*. The central premise of this book is that the intersectionality of diverse skill sets allows for optimum results through brainstorming (Johansson, 2004). It appears that NHS Scotland is stifling such potential through a lack of staff consistency.

### Public Inquiry Findings

For the past few years, the Scottish Government has been holding a public inquiry into the failings of their flagship hospital when it comes to the deaths of four patients through bacterial infections and the contraction of these infections by other patients, especially children on the QEUH children's oncology wards. The latest paper released in 2023, titled; *Provisional Position Paper 5: The History of Infection Concerns (HOIC) for the Queen Elizabeth University Hospital Campus* examines the problems around the cause of the infections. Despite numerous findings, for example, the ignoring of a doctor's concerns over mould spores in a paediatric transplant room, I have decided to focus on the concerns surrounding the waterborne bacteria found in the taps and drains in the wards.

Before the hospital had opened its doors, the infection control doctor (ICD) had raised fears about the ventilation system "particularly in relation to the Adult BMT [bone marrow transplant] unit, the Paediatric BMT Unit and the Infectious Disease Unit" (Scottish Hospitals Inquiries, 2023, p. 7). Concerns, at this time, had also been raised about the taps that had been installed in the hospital, as these were not compliant with NHS Scotland standards. The main worry was over the fitting of flow regulators to the taps, as these had been found to have been the cause of a series of waterborne bacterial infections in neonatal units in Northern Ireland in 2012. At the time of installing the taps, two solutions were proposed: the taps were installed without the flow regulators, and compliant taps were sourced and installed. In the end, the taps were fitted with the flow regulators, which had the added problem in that "[t]he taps which were installed were not compatible with the use of silver hydrogen peroxide, which was to be used in the commissioning process to sanitise the water system" (Scottish Hospitals Inquiries, 2023, p. 8). Prior to the hospital opening, the water system was regularly tested for signs of Legionella. Unfortunately, the testing was carried out by "two F&E [facilities and estates] managers with no training in taking samples" and when some areas tested positive for the bacteria, they simply sanitised the areas they were taken from until three negative tests were given (Scottish Hospitals Inquiries, 2023, p. 8).

There have been several inquiries into the outbreak of infections. In 2018 NHSGGC commissioned Dr Susanne Lee, a consultant clinical scientist, to investigate problems with the water system. Dr Lee concluded that:

> [i]t is likely that the system was contaminated before handover and that fluctuations in the water temperature experienced since opening of the hospital were also a likely contributing factor; and that fungus in the water system was likely due to the dust levels around the site during construction and demolitions. (Scottish Hospitals Inquiries, 2023, p. 39).

In September 2018, it was announced that some of the children's wards were to be closed to allow for a deep cleaning of the wards, the ventilation system, and drains. Despite the deep clean in February 2019, three water samples tested positive for Legionella. Regular testing continued throughout the coming year, with the taps finally being changed in March 2019. Fungus was still evident in the water tanks in June 2019, with water not being declared "pristine" (2023, p. 86) until November of that year. The Scottish Hospital Inquiries have reported that:

> contamination of the water system was thought to have occurred one or more times during installation, and that best practice had not been followed in the design, installation, handover, operation, or maintenance of the water system. (2023, p. 67).

It is not as if any of these concerns had not been raised over the years. As early as September 2017, three consultant microbiologists had begun an official whistleblowing procedure. They raised concerns about "issues with ventilation, a lack of information about commissioning and validation, issues with the water system and concerns about water testing" (2023, p. 28). Yet it appears that not much was done to alleviate their worries.

In 2019, Health Improvement Scotland carried out an unannounced inspection of the QEUH. As part of their report, they noted aspects that NHSGGC could improve on. One thing that needed resolving was staff shortages of both nursing and domestic staff. The inspectors were informed that there was "a 14.5% absence and 10% vacancy rate for domestic staff" (2019, p.8). Added to the problem of staff shortages was a less than satisfactory working relationship between the infection control team and the F&E department. These problems were caused by F&E management not taking on board concerns raised by the infection control team concerning the cleaning of vent ducts, and "not taking on board the concerns of clinical staff during estates meetings." (2019, p. 8). The pressure the domestic staff were under to keep the hospital clean was also highlighted. Not only were staff using the wrong or wrong strength chemicals to clean wash basins, etc, but there were simply not enough mop heads to go around with the domestic supervisor saying that they had never been made aware of the problem (2019, p. 19). Poor communication can, once again, be seen to be placing patients at risk of iatrogenic harm.

The final outcome from all the inquiries appears to be the usual aphorism *lessons will be learnt.* Yet, the NHSGGC may not have gotten off with just a slap on the wrists as the public awoke on the 12th of November 2023 to headlines in the media such as "Scotland's largest health board a formal suspect in corporate homicide investigation." (Johnson, 2023). This could pave the way for the prosecution of senior management.

**Complaining: patients and families**

We discussed in Chapter Three the problems NHS staff encounter when raising concerns about unsafe staffing levels, whether they direct complaints to management or through whistleblowing. In this section I will look at the problems patients and their families experience when attempting to hold the NHS to account. Despite its prevalence within British culture, complaining has negative connotations, with complainers being given nicknames such as *Disgusted of Tunbridge Wells, whiner,* or, in present times, *Karen*[11] Complaining can alienate people, this is especially true if one is a serial complainer. It can also have a negative psychological effect in that it enhances negative emotions. This happens as:

> [t]he human brain, geared for survival, focuses on negatives (as they appear more threatening to survival) than on positives (which enhance life but are less vital for survival). As the brain perceives negatives at an approximated ratio of five to one, there is simply more to complain about than there is to be grateful for. (Berry, 2021).

This can lead to an overall greater feeling of sadness or despondency. Conversely, there are positive effects of complaining, especially when one is doing so vocally, all of which I benefited from: see Introduction. Firstly, you can connect to others with similar experiences. Secondly, complaining by venting allows one to gain an external perspective to the situation and can be viewed as self-monitoring. It enables one to consider if these feelings are justified or not. Is the experience being blown out of all proportion, or are these emotions acceptable? Finally, if the complaint is upheld or if others have similar experiences, it can give a sense of validation (Berry, 2021).

Although the government has made specific changes to their systems to encourage people to complain as part of their patient safety protocols, I argue that a *culture of silence* continues. Sirrs notes that people may still struggle to make complaints as "patients could find the complaints procedures confusing and difficult to navigate" (Sirrs, 2023, p.3). NHS Scotland's Patients' Charter "gives patients a right to give feedback and make comments and raise concerns or complaints about the care they have received" (Scottish Government, 2022). Following his daughter, Molly, contracting a bacterial infection at the QEUH whilst undergoing cancer treatment, Professor John Cuddihy, raised concerns about the cause of the infection. It was believed the infection came from the

---

[11] Disgusted of Tunbridge Wells is a term used to describe an individual of a conservative nature who writes letters of complaint to newspapers in moral outrage with something they disagree with. There are disputes over where this term came from but Disgusted is the pseudonym of the letter writer and Tunbridge Wells, a town in Kent, is where they reside.

hospital environment. Following the complaint, the communications director of NHSGGC, Sandra Bustillo, is said to have told her staff, "a concerned parent may have 'won the battle but won't win the war'" (Aitkin, 2023). This rhetoric shows blatant contempt by QEUH management when it comes to the regard in which they hold patients and their families. This exchange with staff only came to light after a whistleblower, who has since left the QEUH, went to the Scottish press; stating, "I didn't join the NHS to go to war with families (Aitkin, 2023). Interestingly, only one part of Professor Cuddihy's complaint was upheld and that was poor communication with families with reference to the remarks made by Ms. Bustillo.

To assist with communication between patients and the NHS, individuals could be encouraged to fill out patient satisfaction survey forms. This would give management an oversight of not only negative concerns re care but also highlight the much-overlooked positive experiences. Positive feedback can help foster an environment of positivity and increase staff morale. These forms are available in all health care settings as they are viewed as being "an integral element of patient-centred care" (Gilmore et al. 2023, p. 1). Despite their wide use, Gilmore et al. note that the information gleaned from the forms is not being used to its best advantage. The data used is very localised and any initiatives that are started are not fully evaluated. Gilmore et al. propose that not only should any initiatives be fully documented and reviewed locally but that "[l]ongitudinal studies of such initiatives would be useful to better understand how to improve patient experience" (2023, p. 8).

Both Roseanne and I complained to NHSGGC about the treatment our mums were given. I began by visiting NHS Scotland's website and found the email address to lodge my complaint. I complained about the care in the hospital and the time spent waiting for an ambulance. I received an email reply, approximately ten days later, saying that I had sent the email to the wrong department, and I was given another email address. I forwarded the complaints, and after another week or so, I received an email saying that this was no longer the correct department, and I was furnished with a third email address. I waited for another week and then received an email saying that they would look into the hospital complaint, but the ambulance complaint would have to be sent to another department. After about a month or two, I received emails regarding both complaints saying there was no fault to be found in the care my mum received, but I could take it further by writing to the Scottish Public Services Ombudsman. I decided to take that route. I had a reply within a week stating that I would be allocated a case worker, but that would take around ten months. I replied, thanking them for the update and signing it, for the first time, **Dr** Yvonne Bennett. I had a case worker call me within the week to inform me they had been allocated by case; I also receive updates every two weeks. On the 22nd of August 2023, I received a full report regarding the hospital complaint, which stated, "your complaint has not been taken further" the ombudsman has decided not to instigate a full investigation. As I write this chapter, we have not heard any more about the ambulance complaint. This has been held up as the ombudsman has had difficulty getting the relevant paperwork and information from the Scottish Ambulance Service.[12]

Roseanne and her family had similar problems when complaining and this part of her story gave us the opportunity to analyse how individuals "engage in meaningful social action within the constraints of their particular cultural and historical contexts" (Maine, Pierce and Laslett, 2008, p. 133). They also wanted their mum's death certificate altered and to have COVID-19 removed as a cause of death. The QEUH are stating that Roseanne's mum removed the oxygen tubing from her mask, something the family strongly dispute. Following her death, when the family were in their mum's room saying their goodbyes, Roseanne's brother attempted to remove the tubing from the mask and had great difficulty in doing so. As was mentioned earlier, Jean's hands were crippled with arthritis; she could not even do up her buttons, so would have been unable to grip the tubing. The family contacted the procurator fiscal to ask for a post-mortem to be carried out as they felt the death was sudden, unexplained, and suspicious. Their request was denied. After three months, the family were eventually called to a meeting at the hospital, they were surprised that the investigation into their mum's care was being carried out by the hospital itself. They were also told there was no cause for complaint and directed to the ombudsman. The family then had the same reply from the ombudsman as I had; their complaint had not been upheld. Roseanne has also employed the media to get her mum's story heard, she has been on Scottish Television (STV) news and in the newspapers. Age Concern became involved due to the pressure Roseanne was under to place a DNR order. After they had exhausted all avenues, the family turned to a lawyer. They were charged £5000 to have their mum's notes sent to the law firm. Unfortunately, there was not enough evidence to progress with a negligence claim. Her mum's observation charts were all in order, something Roseanne strongly disputes as she was with her mum for a lot of the time and states that observations were not being carried out for two hours as stated in the notes. It became a *he said, she said*

---

[12] Just before this book went to print, I received an email informing me that the complaint against the Scottish Ambulance Service had not been upheld as my mum's injury was not life threatening/ changing. This is despite research showing that 50% of elderly who are left lying on the floor for over two hours die within 12 months (Khraief, Benzarti and Amiri, 2020). Sadly, my mum is another statistic that can be added to that data, dying seven months after her accident. I finally received an apology form the Scottish Ambulance Service two years after my mum's accident.

situation. Although Tracy raised a complaint at ward level about the nurse, she did not make a formal complaint about her dad's care as "you don't get anywhere" (Tracy, 2022).

Roseanne and I thought that obstacles were placed in our way to stop us from complaining. Our perception was that if we were given, *the run around,* we would eventually give up. From the outset of this research project, we were aware that all our participants had their own reasons for agreeing to take part. Maines, Pierce and Laslett wrote that the motivation for some narrators may simply be the opportunity to get a hearing (2008, p. 111), and this was indeed the prime motivation for all our participants as for too long they felt their complaints and concerns had fallen on deaf ears.

With the increasing numbers of elderly and their greater use of the NHS, the Parliamentary and Health Service Ombudsman produced a paper that looked at the barriers the elderly face when making complaints about the NHS. They found that there were four main reasons why the elderly do not make complaints:

- Lack of information on how to complain and who to direct the complaint to.

- Do not like to make a fuss and worry about the consequences of doing so.

- Believe it will make no difference.

- Do not have support in helping them with the complaint (2015, p. 2).

Realising there was a need to assist the elderly in the complaints process the ombudsman proposed that support and information needed to be specifically targeted towards the elderly via an advocacy service. With only a quarter of all complaints, at this present time, coming from those aged 65 years and older, it is important that such services are initiated, or we risk alienating the elderly from the complaints procedure altogether.

# Chapter Six

# **Connecting the Fragments**

## Christina Stead

### Introduction

According to Finch, Wilson and Bibby's (2023) report for the Health Foundation "the health of the population is one of any nation's greatest assets" p. 16), yet, as research continues to report, it appears that Scotland is failing to protect and capitalise on that precious asset. In the preceding chapters, we have discussed the challenges faced by the NHS at the time of writing in 2023/24. Our analysis has examined the situation facing NHS Scotland, with a particular focus on Glasgow, the location of our ethnographic study. Before the final chapter of the book takes a reflexive review of the research, the focus of this chapter returns to the themes already discussed, connecting them to wider research to explore the extent to which our findings are supported by other studies and also setting them in the context of the national policy agenda. This serves to connect the research to the wider context - where the personal meets the political, as Wright Mills (1959) would have it. The broader policy environment is first considered, showing how policies of austerity, emanating from the Westminster government, set the framework for Scotland as a whole and Glasgow in particular. Attention then moves to the NHS and the very particular relationship between this public service and the British public, who fund it via taxation and use (and sometimes misuse) its services. Lastly, we examine a key theme we derived from our data, namely the difficulties that participants have in communicating with clinical staff.

### The Political Effect: Austerity

*Austerity, n Sternness or severity of manner, appearance, or disposition; severity in judgement... harshness, severity (OED 2023)*

As a result of the 2007 financial crash, policies of austerity were followed, initially by the Labour government and then, from 2010, the Conservative-

Liberal Democrat coalition government.[1] Put simply, there was a reduction in government spending to control levels of public sector debt. In the UK, this resulted in the loss of 490,000 public sector jobs, a 19% reduction in the budget, the raising of the retirement age from age 65 to 66, a reduction in the income tax allowance for pensioners, and cuts to child benefits. The purpose of these measures was to encourage investment and return a positive national balance sheet. There was no political will to levy higher taxes. Economic policies of austerity have wide consequences, for society more broadly and for health services. For Stuckler et al. (2017, p.18), austerity represented "a massive experiment", the effects of which have disproportionately affected the most vulnerable groups in society. As explained above, some austerity measures specifically targeted elderly people and children. Reductions in public spending in areas such as housing or health have adversely impacted the safety nets designed to protect the vulnerable. Furthermore, cuts to one area go on to affect others: for example, homelessness will place additional pressure on health services because a lack of shelter brings greater risk to personal safety and exposure to illness, often leading to poor health. This is in addition to other disadvantages, such as access to employment opportunities. Food insecurity/ poverty is now commonly experienced, and queues at local food banks are a regular sight even in the affluent commuter belt in southern England. Poverty and disadvantage also lead to poor mental health, with, for example, job loss, underemployment, or lack of access to *good work* being associated with depression. For the elderly, the primary focus of this book, austerity measures have had an adverse effect on mortality. McCartney et al. note that austerity policies are "highly likely to be the most substantial causal contributor to stalled mortality trends seen in Scotland" (2022, p.52). Our participants told stories that set individual lives in the context of policy decisions: this is where narrative offers Wright Mills' (1959) bridge between the personal and the political.

In addition to the personal effects of austerity, policies have had a broader impact. For example, research by Fetzer (2019) has suggested that significant links can be made between the adoption of austerity policies and the outcome of the 2016 referendum when the UK voted to leave the European Union. Specifically, the Vote Leave campaign picked up broader dissatisfactions felt by communities that had been adversely affected by austerity policies. NHS funding was used, with a key image of the campaign suggesting that the UK's

---

[1] The election held on 6th May 2010 saw a swing to the Conservative party, however, they were 20 seats short of an overall majority so there was a hung parliament. The party entered into a coalition government with the Liberal Democrat party that lasted until the general election of 7th May 2015, won by the Conservatives with a majority of 10 seats.

contribution to the EU budget could instead be spent on healthcare services. Fetzer (2019) also suggests a correlation between support for the United Kingdom Independence Party (UKIP) and geographical districts badly affected by austerity policies.[2] The financial effects of Brexit are yet to be fully manifested, and this is highly likely to be an area of keen interest for future researchers.

Since its establishment in 1948, the NHS has continued to enjoy general support from the public (Burkitt et al., 2018). This has continued throughout the years of austerity policies, and its status as a priority area for public funding continues unabated. The relationship is, however, complex. As an illustration, public discourse around the NHS and its constituent services is often emotive and, as noted in the Introduction to this book, this can translate into lurid media headlines such as that describing what happened to Dr Bennett's mother: "Glasgow great-gran endured five hours 'screaming in agony' on care home floor waiting on ambulance" (McGill and Duffy, 2022). Another aspect of the emotional response was on display in the Thursday evening *Clap for the NHS* sessions that ran for ten weeks during the 2020 lockdown in the UK. The purpose of the initiative was to allow the public to show support for front-line workers, and it seems to have acted as a communal outlet at a time when other social activities were banned. It is notable that the Royal College of Nursing, representing the profession, did not support a proposed return of the weekly round of applause, stating that nurses did not want to be seen as heroes and that the public could best show its support for the NHS by complying with COVID-19 precautions (Mitchell, 2021). Media headlines speak of the British public *falling out of love* with the NHS, suggesting a quasi-romantic relationship with what is, in reality, a complex public company (Stewart, 2023). Such stories imply that the NHS as an organisation, or its constituent services, are somehow one large amorphous mass and that public opinion is divided along binary lines of love or hate, ignorant of nuance. Healthcare is an intensely personal issue, yet individual stories, such as those of Jean, John or Ella, are easily lost in the wider context of funding or policy. Equally, Jordan's and Sam's experiences of work are worthy of illumination and add further perspective to headline figures of staff shortages or ambulance waiting times. Whilst this book also examines broader issues, it was conceived to ensure that our participants and their stories would not simply be seen as numbers in statistical data. The next section will review the national situation in Scotland before issues specific to the city of Glasgow are considered.

---

[2] UKIP was the principal party campaigning to leave the European Union (EU).

## The Scotland Effect

Throughout the book, we have provided socio-economic and health data to enable the reader to connect our participants' narratives to the broader context. This guards against the fragmentation of stories and connects them to the wider framework within which our participants have lived and worked (West, 1996). Since devolution in 1999, the Scottish government has set the fiscal and policy agenda for NHS Scotland, allocating public money, and managing the service. (Note that this, however, comes within the UK-wide decision to pursue the measures of austerity described earlier in this chapter.) Despite clear policy intent, data show that in the last two decades, health inequalities have increased. A key evaluation report from the Health Foundation, *Leave No one Behind* (Finch, Wilson and Bibby, 2023), describes public services as "fragile" (p.7) and notes that, whilst there is evidence of policy ambition to improve the health of the people of Scotland, implementation has been ineffective. As the report unequivocally states, 'joined-up policy design and delivery matters' (p. 2). In earlier chapters, we have noted the challenges thrown up by the 2007 financial crisis, the 2019 COVID-19 pandemic and the current cost-of-living crisis. All have conspired to send measures of health improvement into reverse: for example, after a period of improvement, levels of excess mortality in Glasgow have begun to increase. There is a pressing need to secure coherence of policy between government, sectors (such as health and social care services or charity) and local areas, and also for timely and strong evaluations of effectiveness. These measures need to be taken to promote a sustained and long-term approach to health improvement across society and to protect current and future vulnerabilities in the interests of improved social consequences (Finch, Wilson and Bibby, 2023).

The same report (Finch, Wilson and Bibby, 2023) highlights the crisis faced by NHS Scotland because of the convergence of long-term inequalities with short-term misuse of services. Whilst there are clear challenges in Scotland throughout the life course, the ageing population presents additional and pressing issues to health and social care services (Elston et al., 2019; Leith and Sim, 2022). The proportion of elderly people is increasing at a faster rate than those aged 15 or under, and the government estimates that, by 2039, 800,000 people will be over the age of 75 (Scottish Government 2023). Although the population taken as a whole is ageing, life expectancy in Scotland is the lowest of the four nations of the United Kingdom. Data are notably lower for those living in the most deprived areas of the country. The gap between years of healthy life expectancy for the richest and poorest in society has been increasing since 2016, that is, before the effects of the pandemic had been felt, such that Scotland now faces issues brought about by:

a toxic combination of adverse historical living conditions and waves of detrimental national and local government policymaking which have resulted in a greater vulnerability of the population to the effects of other, well-understood, political, and social determinants of health. (Walsh et al. 2021, p.1199).

## The Glasgow Effect

The situation described above is bleak across Scotland, but it is particularly acute in Glasgow, the location of this study. The city is statistically significant for the nation as a whole, with the wider metropolitan area representing approximately 31% of the population and the City of Glasgow 11% (National Records for Scotland, 2022). For the World Health Organisation, the main drivers of health inequalities continue to be socio-economic (Wilkinson and Marmot, 2003). Particular circumstances conspire to jeopardise the health of Glaswegians, so research has sought to understand exactly why Glasgow suffers from high levels of excess mortality, especially when compared to areas of the UK with a similar deprivation index, such as the cities of Liverpool, Manchester or Belfast. Walsh et al. (2016) evaluated different hypotheses for this bleak picture, including economic, social and environmental factors. The research examined the wide range of suggested indicators, including disadvantage and poverty; the effects of deindustrialisation; the wealth gap between the richest and poorest districts; historically overcrowded, poor quality and poorly maintained housing; the consequences of the new towns planning approach of the 1960s and 70s with its socially selective policy of relocating certain sectors of the population outside the city centre; sectarianism; and low levels of access to higher education and consequentially lower attainment (Walsh et al. 2016). Most of the hypotheses were found to be credible, with some (e.g. disadvantage and poverty) considered especially strong. Since that research was published in 2016, the situation has worsened, and a recent evaluation shows that health inequalities across the whole of Scotland are increasing because the effects of structural inadequacies (such as those described above) have been exacerbated by further crisis points, such as the 2007 financial crash or, more recently, the COVID-19 pandemic and cost of living crisis. These exposed what is described as the *societal fault line* and have left the most disadvantaged sectors of the population continuing to experience the worst outcomes in relation to health (Finch, Wilson and Bibby, 2023). Whenever health issues are suffered by the Scottish population as a whole, it appears that Glasgow feels the most acute effects. Those effects are not, however, distributed equally throughout the population, so it would be wrong to suggest a homogeneously bleak scenario as Glasgow also has pockets of extreme wealth, such as the suburb of Bearsden or the affluent West End districts. Indeed, the wealth gap between the richest and the poorest in Glasgow is significant and continues to increase. According to the Glasgow Indicators Project (2023), 32% of children in the city were living in poverty in 2021-22, perhaps also a reflection of the fact that the salaries of the 20% highest earners are more than double the pay of the lowest 20% of employees. The highest disparity in child poverty was between Govanhill (70%) and West End areas like Carmunock (below 5%).

In addition to the picture described above, the population of Scotland, but especially Glasgow, suffers from greater vulnerability to deaths caused by the so-called *diseases of despair* namely alcohol or drug misuse and suicide, with middle-aged men originally being particularly affected. Earlier in the book, Dr Bennett discussed the high rates of suicide amongst male paramedics; for some time, male suicide has been a recognised phenomenon, attracting attention from researchers and policymakers and leading to publications such as the Scottish Government's *Every Life Matters – Scotland's Suicide Prevention Action Plan* (2018). Data is now, however, indicating that an increased number of women are dying as a result of alcohol, drugs or suicide; for example, Walsh et al. (2021) found that between 2015 and 2017, more women were dying of drug poisoning in Scotland than in England and Wales combined. In terms of alcohol-related deaths, the Scottish Government's policy on minimum alcohol pricing, introduced in 2018, is failing to have the desired effects. Wyper et al. reported a socio-economic pattern in that alcohol-related deaths are "over five times higher, in the most, compared with the least deprived areas" (2023, p. 1361). These statistics are a further indication of the worsening picture of health for the population of Glasgow.

This review of national and local indicators clearly shows that the lifespan of an individual is affected by interlinking determinants. This returns the analysis squarely to the urgent need for effective and sustained policy, implementation, and monitoring. I now turn to the issue of the provision of health services within Glasgow, first explaining how NHS Scotland is feeling the adverse effects of a cut in the number of nurse training places.

Within Scotland, there has been opposition to austerity policies, with the SNP, the majority party, denouncing them as *cruel*. A key platform for the party continues to be the 'will to mitigate mistakes', as campaigning material puts it (2022). So how, then, have health services been affected by austerity? Sam and several of the TikTok respondents spoke of the deleterious impact on the recruitment, retention, and morale of staff. There is also an impact on patient safety, via increased risk of iatrogenic harm, as Dr Bennett discussed in an earlier chapter. Jeffries et al.'s report for the Nuffield Trust (2023) suggests that a 2011 decision to cut nurse training places has now led to chronic shortages across the UK, despite government assurances to the contrary at the time [3], the decision was apparently based on a government estimation that there would be an oversupply of trained nurses, leading to consequent unemployment.[4] The cuts were described as a ticking time bomb by a senior academic nurse (Quallington, 2015) in an opinion piece in the *Health Services Journal*. This claim was then strongly refuted by Health Education England, which, in direct response to Quallington's comments, confirmed that the aim was to prevent unemployment for members of the nursing profession. Whilst financial support is available to nursing students in Scotland, levels of recruitment have not recovered, and 2023 statistics show that 11.8% of NHS nursing vacancies remain unfilled, representing a record-high percentage (nurses.co.uk, 2023). As a large hospital, the QEUH suffers from the practical effects of nursing under-recruitment. When it opened in the spring of 2015, it was the flagship part of a wider health strategy intended to address fiscal issues by concentrating services on one site to make efficiency gains alongside cutting-edge clinical excellence that would bring benefits to the health of the local population. As this book has explained, these intentions have not yet been effectively delivered, as evidenced by the ongoing public inquiry into problems arising from environmental and construction defects, issues stemming from the design of the building, such as the use of single rooms, and the difficulties caused by the lift system, mentioned by several of our participants. In addition to the well-documented design and construction concerns, our research found direct evidence of the effects of staffing shortages. Although not working specifically in elderly care, in their narrative, Sam described the effects of shortages on the morale and health of nursing staff at QEUH and these cannot solely be attributed to the pandemic, albeit that those exceptional circumstances exacerbated existing challenges. In response, the Scottish Government launched a nursing and midwifery task force in February 2023 to improve working conditions and boost retention, however, this comes at a time when recruitment to undergraduate nursing courses in Scotland is declining and, in elderly care, vacancies have never been higher (RCN, 2023).

Care of the elderly forms part of all adult nursing preregistration programmes, but it does not generally appear to be taught as discrete content. Whilst this is understandable, in that elderly patients will present with the same conditions as people at earlier stages of the lifespan, and that it would not be appropriate or desirable to isolate them further, it does imply that there are no specialised clinical needs and may also reflect a feeling that nursing the elderly may be a

---

[4] Anne Milton, then the Health Minister, explained that the cuts were necessary to prevent an oversupply of nurses in the workplace.

lower-status role than other specialities. Yet, as Age Concern notes, "the health and social care system is not yet equipped to deal with the challenges that an ageing population brings" (2023, p.36).[5] In Scotland, this currently translates to vacancy levels in elderly social care running at 64% (RCN, 2023), though, as discussed in Chapter Four, the Scottish government provides free care to all elderly people over 65 years of age who need assistance, hence the workforce required is proportionally much larger per head of population than that in, say, England. I looked at online prospectuses for four randomly selected undergraduate nursing programmes at the University of the West of Scotland (2023), Hertfordshire University (2023), Glasgow Caledonian University (2023) and Northumbria University (2023) and could find no references in the marketing material to care of the elderly. Course webpages instead tended to highlight career opportunities in areas such as palliative care, oncology or intensive care, fields that are deemed to appeal more powerfully to prospective nursing students. Given the rising proportion of elderly people within the general population, the challenges of staffing elderly care are likely to become ever more acute, so the establishment of the nursing and midwifery task force is timely. At its congress in 2023, the RCN passed a resolution calling for the appointment of a commissioner for older people, a further indication of a shift in policy.

When at QEUH with her mother, Dr Bennett observed different types of staffing problems. The consolidation of services onto one hospital site had led to the creation of large teams, such as was the case in radiography where even managers were unfamiliar with their colleagues and uncertain of their capabilities or training needs. Heavy reliance on agency nurses created a lack of continuity of care and wasted resources as, in addition to high agency fees, precious nursing time had to be used as they were inducted into ward routines and practices. It should be noted that the NHS will also have provided training placements and funding for many of these nurses. Sam reported that nurses were bussed into the QEUH from elsewhere to cover shortages, presumably with negative effects on their home healthcare facilities. From within the Scottish Ambulance Service, Jordan reported that paramedics were suffering similar stressors, leading to burn-out and defection to private ambulance providers. All these are the consequences of political decisions made at national and regional levels and, again, serve as stark reminders of the collision between the political and the personal.

## Misuse of the NHS

Yet problems in health services do not begin and end with managers and staff. Whilst the general public has generally high expectations of the NHS, it is clear

---

[5] Age Concern is a UK-based charity advocating for the needs of the elderly population.

that patients should play their part in using its constituent services in a timely and appropriate fashion. Behaviours such as missing appointments, avoidable attendance at emergency departments or the misuse of ambulance services all conspire to place greater strain on resources, with consequently deleterious effects for future patients. As noted by the Health Foundation, if Scotland's current position with regard to health and health inequalities is to improve, the public must play its part (Finch, Wilson and Bibby, 2023). In Chapter Three, we discussed Jordan's dispiriting experiences as a paramedic working for the Scottish Ambulance Service and both Dr Bennett and Tracy reported the distressing effects of excessive ambulance waiting times on their ill, elderly parents. In Chapter Three, the phenomenon of ambulance so-called frequent fliers – people who repeatedly misuse the service - was discussed. Research by the King's Fund (Burkett et al. 2018), commissioned to examine public perceptions of the NHS at 70, explored the notion of a deal between the public and the health service, in that certain expectations should be placed on both partners so that whilst the former should undertake not to misuse services, the latter needed to communicate more effectively and operate more efficiently. The issue of communication certainly chimes with our research. From one perspective, it is clear that better signposting of services could help patients access the right service at the right time and thereby bring benefits such as reduced pressure on emergency and acute services. This would, however, require patients to feel confident of securing appointments in the primary care system, such as with GP practices. Since the pandemic, however, practices have been under severe strain (Finch, Wilson and Bibby, 2023). As is true of hospital-based nurses, following the pandemic, primary care staff are also at risk of burnout as a result of stress. GP vacancies are also running at high levels.

## Communication with Health Services Staff

Where staff are over-stretched and working in the suboptimal environment that our research suggests is the case at the QEUH, patients are less likely to receive high-quality care. The narratives in this book raise issues of significance around poor communication between health service staff, patients, and their family members. Communication is one of the Nursing and Midwifery Council's most important competencies for nurses (NMC, 2018), and communication and other so-called soft skills are now routinely taught to medical students and in other clinical training programmes. Despite this, both Tracy and Roseanne reported incidents where clinicians had not communicated effectively, Roseanne in response to a request that the family agree to a DNR notice and Tracy when she queried her father's oxygen levels and also formally reported a serious problem with unauthorised access to her father when he was in hospital. Perceptions of effective communication are subjective and will be affected by emotional responses; the situations described by our participants were indeed emotionally challenging, and it should also be recognised that the clinicians in question were navigating the exceptional circumstances of the COVID-19 pandemic. Whilst good communication carries strong benefits and should be a minimum requirement of modern-day healthcare, our research (even with the pandemic caveat above) illuminates the lasting damage to families when it falls short.

Our findings also emphasise the importance of timely communication for patients and their families. Roseanne explained the difficulties and frustrations of trying to contact the staff who were caring for her mother, saying that she had telephoned over 50 times without success. When eventually she did get through to the ward, nobody called her back. This is something that I have also experienced, though, eventually, the use of my doctoral title led to rapid action. Whilst it must be acknowledged that clinical situations can change quickly and that staff are under pressure for the reasons discussed throughout this book, both Roseanne and Tracy reported having been given contradictory information about their respective parent's condition. Tracy raised a formal complaint with the QEUH after an incident where an estranged family member was told to come to her dying father's bedside despite instructions to the contrary in his medical notes. As reported in Chapter Four, effective communication is of paramount importance when it concerns DNR notices: whilst, understandably, they are often required in emergencies, our research concurs with that of Bows and Herring (2022) and Tomkow et al. (2023) in that both Roseanne and Dr Bennett were contacted unexpectedly by telephone and asked to agree to a DNR being placed on their parent. The women reached different conclusions but shared disquiet at what they had been asked to do. The issues around DNR notices are complex; for example, they may also reflect a broader reluctance to confront mortality, as reported by Cherniak (2002) but, if an informed decision is to be made, then relatives must be given sufficient information and, ideally, time to evaluate choices.

This returns the analysis to Dr Bennett's discussion in the previous chapter around patient-centred care (PCC) and the conflict with medical paternalism. The latter phenomenon is seen when patients (or, we would argue, families) are not deemed to have sufficient autonomy to make effective decisions and could certainly be applied to both Roseanne's experience with the DNR order and Tracy's with the admission of the unauthorised family member to her dying father's bedside. Autonomy is deemed to be a fundamental part of medical ethics; however, the issue is complex, and it is suggested that the notion of the best interests of a patient extends beyond solely medical interests (Foster 2019). Both Tracy and Roseanne reported feeling powerless in the face of the medical establishment whilst trying to advocate for their parents:

- It had been written down how distressed my dad had been when he saw her. He [the nurse] told me it was her right to know. (Tracy, 2022).

- The doctors were insisting I sign the DNR, and when I once again refused was told they would take it out of my hands and put one in place. (Roseanne, 2023).

Notions of what constitutes good communication are subjective, and Roseanne and Tracy were reporting on particularly difficult and emotionally-charged incidents, however, whilst clinical staff are now given specific training, the effects of mis- or inept communication can have significant effects. Our participants found themselves returning to these interactions and were still upset by them nearly two years later.

## Conclusions

By 2050, 1:6 people in Scotland will be aged 65 or over, and the challenges discussed in this book will only grow larger. In common with every nation, Scotland needs to be ready to support its elderly. Our data and other research have highlighted the particular challenges faced in Glasgow. Statistical data on health are already alarming, and trends, such as excess mortality rates, are only worsening. Health policy sits in the wider context of austerity and strained public finances, however, the consequences of failing to address health issues will be even more costly. Whilst the public has a right to expect an effective service, individuals must play their part in using the NHS properly. There are practical responsibilities, like the need to avoid calling ambulances unnecessarily or to keep appointments; individuals also hold some responsibility for their health and the impact that behavioural choices will have.

The scale of health inequalities in Scotland is such that there is no easy fix. In its report *Leave No one Behind* (Finch, Wilson and Bibby, 2023), the Health Foundation is clear that there needs to be an improvement in policy delivery and coordination to prevent replication of effort and to ensure that public funds are spent effectively and with due accountability. Many of the issues identified through the research reported in this book would not be unique to Glasgow, as NHS services throughout the country face similar constraints and challenges: indeed, I can attest to significant problems of communication and staffing in an English hospital that treated a member of my family. In Glasgow, the QEUH is charged with delivering healthcare to one of the most disadvantaged populations in Western Europe in one of the most modern hospitals in the UK. Huge resources have been invested in the fabric of the building, yet it has been beset with problems, environmental and social. Our participants also reported concerns with clinical practice that have been pursued through formal channels of complaint, albeit with some difficulty. Whilst it is not appropriate to comment on the specific health conditions of their relatives, it does appear that the design of the building – particularly the use of single bedrooms for all patients – might not be fit for purpose. This is especially relevant to the care of the elderly, where social interaction is so valuable. Taken together, health policy and the health care that is subsequently offered within the policy framework, perhaps represent the ultimate collision of the political with the personal.

As discussed in this chapter, the NHS continues to enjoy broad support from the public despite well-documented problems, most notably staff shortages. Funding continues to be challenging, and the ongoing effects of austerity policies on public health place a further strain on services. The situation is particularly acute in Scotland and especially in Glasgow, reflected in the 300,000 responses to Yvonne Bennett's TikTok post about healthcare struggles. The NHS is a hugely beneficial resource. It should be funded properly, managed effectively and used wisely.

The research reported in this book was not specifically conceived to develop the health policy agenda, however analysis of the participants' stories suggests a number of measures that might be taken to improve the experiences of patients and staff alike.

### Suggestions to alleviate pressure on the NHS:

- Geriatric care specialists, this field of medicine should be actively promoted to give appropriate recognition to clinical and social care professionals.

- An increase in nursing staff across all bands. This should begin with additional student places at the university, supported by appropriate funding arrangements.

- To help to retain staff, bullying must be handled properly with all complaints taken seriously. Audits were carried out on lecturers and mentors of all student nurses. Student nurse, placement review forms are to be given credence and not viewed as grievance outlets.

- Further investment in mental health hubs for all NHS staff.

- To decrease pressure on emergency and acute NHS services, funding should be directed at minor injury units, pharmacies and GP practices, with appropriate information signposting campaigns.

- Expertise within clinical fields, including nursing, should be recognized as part of a career progression to management.

- Although highly problematic in operational and ethical terms, consideration should be given to levying sanctions on people who regularly miss appointments.

- At present, some NHS services (e.g. accident and emergency treatment) are free to all, regardless of domicile or nationality. Given the parlous state of NHS finances, this could be reviewed to bring the UK in line with other European nations.

### Suggestions to improve patient satisfaction:

- The complaints system to be streamlined, with an initial designated contact who would then liaise with departmental managers. To resolve complaints, face-to-face meetings would make the process more transparent and may offer closure to complainants.

- Whilst the NHS does collect feedback, the use, analysis and follow-up actions appear inconsistent. Again, this does not encourage transparency or confidence in the process from patients, families or, indeed, staff. Feedback data should be collated, and any resultant local initiatives forwarded to policymakers for assessment and wider adoption as appropriate.

The NHS is a hugely beneficial resource, and, as we have explored throughout this book, it should be funded properly, managed effectively and used wisely. As a large public organization, responsibility for this lies with politicians, staff and patients, for healthcare is where overarching policy, managerial and deeply personal agendas collide. Patient safety should be of paramount importance, however as Sirrs points out, "the NHS still has a long way to go to embody a genuine ethos of patient safety, rather than treating it as a tick box exercise" (2023, p.23).

# Chapter Seven
# **Looking Back to Look Forward**

We have decided to use this concluding chapter as an exercise in reflexivity and reflection. Our choices, from choosing to undertake this research project to using the methodology to finding individual narratives, were analysed at every stage. Throughout we were steadfast that an ethnographic approach using narratives was the optimum methodology. People are, as discussed in Chapter Two, motivated to give meaning to life events and do so through storytelling. It affords them the tools to make sense of experiences, especially those that are traumatic, because "story is a sense-making tool" (Shi, 2021, p. 1).

### **Yvonne**

As reflexivity affords researchers the chance to examine our judgements and opinions, I was compelled to examine my own political beliefs. I was aware that the objective of being reflexive was to identify any personal opinions that may, inadvertently, affect the analysis of data. Could my own bias against the SNP make me prone to leading the data to a certain conclusion? Dr Stead was able to provide the necessary *checks and balances* to my analysis. That being said, by bringing to the table my opinions, my bias, and my experiences, I have ensured that the reader knows where I am in the research. By situating my story with the narratives of the other participants, I was able to extract my life experiences and locate them in the research, both during data collection and analysis. On reflection, I want the readers to know who all of us, who shared our stories, are as individuals. Taking that lead, I am a woman, a sociologist, a Scot, and, perhaps most importantly, my mum's advocate, my mum's voice. These facts have a context in this research, and by acknowledging them through an ethnographic approach, I aimed to be a character in my story and an actor in my research (Katz-Rothman 2007). I am not centre stage, but I am present.

I did not keep a fieldwork diary during the research process, but I was able to rewatch the content I had made on TikTok, and this helped ensure that I could reflect on the narratives that underpin this book. Each participant in this study remained an individual with a history and unique identity; each had a story to tell. Morgan and Guevera (2008) emphasised the importance of the researcher–participant relationship and proposed that "the quality of the research often depends on the quality of the researcher's relationships with the participants" (2008, p. 728). Both Dr Stead and I had connections with the participants be that through being part of the sandwich generation, through our own difficult navigation of the NHS with our elderly parents, or by my connection as a past employee of NHS Scotland. These connections and the rapport established ensured that I was not just another woman who had a traumatic experience and battle with NHS Scotland, and they were not the *objects* in a research project. We were individuals with a common bond.

A major concern I had throughout writing this book was ensuring that we did justice to those whose stories were told. Our goal was to highlight the injustices felt by the participants and to raise awareness of the problems those who use and work in NHS Scotland experience on a daily basis. Shi reported that there is a "positive effect of narrating traumatic experiences in a constructive and purposeful manner" (2021, p. 6).

I did not intend for my own story to have the effect it did, but it became an empathy-inducing story exchange. However, by sharing my story, I not only gave meaning to my traumatic experience, but it also enabled me to better understand others. Our story exchanges fostered empathy an empathy that was easily transferable to the other participants with similar stories to tell. Reflexively, as I look back on this entire experience from August 2022 to the present day, I am of the opinion that we have met our goals, and all our stories have been treated with empathy and respect. As Dr Stead and I wrote this book I sat and watched all the videos, something I found to be both sad and cathartic. Through our voices, we have ensured our parents are more than just a statistic.

### Christina

When I reflect on my reasons for joining the study, I find them to be complex. In my part of the 'Our Stories 'section in Chapter Two, I explained that my situation is different to those of Yvonne and the other participants, in that I am not from Glasgow, a bereaved child or working in NHS Scotland. I live in the South of England and am fortunate that both my parents are still very much alive in their mid-eighties; I have fewer direct personal connections to the research, yet there are some biographical similarities. Yvonne and I met as PhD students and both found that we needed to juggle our research projects alongside the needs of our families, including our parents. My mother had had some health issues and I had battled with parts of the NHS to try to secure satisfactory communication and treatment for her. As a middle aged, highly educated woman who had worked in the public sector, I had been shocked by the difficulty of navigating the system and sought a better understanding of the underlying issues. Whilst Glasgow has its particular problems, documented in this book in unrelenting detail, my own experiences indicate that they are not unique to the city. To return, then, to the point made in Yvonne's reflections above, I am a minor character in the overarching story but have taken a larger role in the overall analysis. I am definitely not centre stage but I, too, am present and my own story has influenced my responses to the participants.

As a social researcher, I am interested in people and their stories: not only the content but also the ways in which they choose to tell them. I do not use TikTok but have accounts on other social media sites and am curious about the choices that all users (including myself) make when deciding how to represent ourselves in what we post, how we react and respond to others, and what all of this might signify. Social media encourages us all to act as performers and there is similarity in the research process when researchers and participants are simultaneously performers and audience. Unlike the other participants, I do not divulge any of the specific details of my mother's story, in (absolutely proper) deference to her wishes but suffice it to say that many of the issues narrated by the participants resonated with me. In Chapter One, we stated that we aimed to produce trustworthy research, and I believe we achieved that by placing our participants' narratives within the literature and data that supports them. As noted in the book, FOI requests were refused and politicians failed to respond or to speak on the record, yet the data that we collected is rich and powerful.

For me, this research speaks primarily of the direct links between policy decisions and individual lives. In Glasgow, the politics of austerity has exacerbated existing socio-economic fault lines and the most disadvantaged in society suffer the effects. Brexit and the COVID-19 pandemic increased the pressure on services that were already overstretched. There are identified causal links between disadvantage and health (McCartney et al., 2022) yet NHS services are expected to pick up the pieces, working under severe resource constraints in a sub-optimal physical environment. The relationship between the public and the NHS is complex, and often contradictory, given that the oft-stated quasi-romantic love for the service sits alongside the evidence of misuse that we have reported.

The raw emotion that was present in all the interviews will stay with me forever; the stories were difficult to hear and challenging to report and represent within the book. Given the issues around the selection and interpretation of data, I have always been wary of claiming to *give voice* to participants, however in this study, it does appear that we have done that. In the final section below, we give the last words to the participants.

## Final Thoughts from the Participants

As the participants remain an integral part of this work, we asked all four to give their reflections. An email was sent to each of them asking why they had wanted to be a part of this book and how they felt now that the book was finally written. As these people were the impetus for the book, we believed the last word should go to them. These are their replies:

**Tracy**

I wanted to do it because I feel like my dad was failed by the NHS, I was given so many different stories on phoning them for updates because we weren't allowed to visit him so was getting positive updates then out of nowhere he was basically dying when a few hours before they said he was sitting up eating soup and I know sometimes that can happen but it was a big shock then to him sitting talking to being totally sedated all in a few hours, I'm glad the book is nearly finished because I feel like I'm being my dad's voice I know so many people aren't being heard on their circumstances,

Thank you so much for giving me the opportunity to be part of your book.

**Sam**

That's great, look forward to reading it.

For me it was just about highlighting the problems in the NHS, the public don't know what goes on in these wards, so it was good to give an insight.

I'm glad I done it and could help highlight some of the issues.

**Jordan**

Your [Yvonne] story in particular made me want to reach out. The overall state of our NHS at the moment, and specifically the issues with the QEUH and the apparent blanket silence of all the issues that have gone on in there, needed brought to light. Your story was one story, that for me as a health professional could have been that of hundreds of people, and really is the same as hundreds of people.

It's a real fear I have for the people of Glasgow, the closures of so many wonderful hospitals, and loss of highly skilled staff members because of the decline in our services, has had such a profound effect on people's care and will only continue as the years go on. Unfortunately, the majority of people's eyes remain closed to the problems faced and they have no interest in hearing, or they swing so far the other way in anger that they can't rationalise or be listened to.

There needed to be a middle ground of honesty and openness and I really can't wait to see the finished product.

**Roseanne**

I wanted to take part in the book because it gives a platform for my mum's story to be heard. I am extremely grateful that I was given this opportunity. The book now being published is a humbling experience as this means that collectively the families involved in this book will shed light on the real day to day of the NHS and the lives being lost.

# Appendix 1

A research study is being conducted by **Dr Yvonne Bennett and Dr Christina Stead**

**This research project is examining the ways in which the elderly are being treated within the Scottish National Health Service with reference to the Queen Elizabeth University Hospital (QEUH), Glasgow.**

## What will you be required to do?

We are looking for volunteers to be interviewed, either on a one-to-one basis or in a small group, about their experiences with the QEUH. The interviews will be semi structured and recorded. All data gathered will be strictly confidential and anonymous. Any removal of anonymity will be at the participants request and will be looked at on a case-to-case basis.

## To participate in this research, you must:

be over 16 years of age.

## Feedback

We will present feedback on a regular basis to each of the participants. This can either be face to face when either of the researchers return to Glasgow, by telephone, by text messaging or private messaging through social media.

All data and personal information will be stored securely in accordance with the Data Protection Act 1998. Data can only be accessed by Yvonne Bennett and Christina Stead.

## Dissemination of results

All results will be published in the book titled *The Stories Behind the Statistics: How the Scottish NHS is letting down the elderly.* Results can be provided on request.

## Deciding whether to participate

If you have any questions or concerns about the nature, procedures or requirements for participation do not hesitate to contact either of us. Should you decide to participate, you will be free to withdraw at any time without having to give a reason.

# Appendix 2

DIRECTORATE FOR HEALTH WORKFORCE

DHWLSR: Pay, Practice and Information Governance

16 November 2023
Dear Yvonne Bennett,

Thank you for your e-mail of 11 October 2023 addressed to Michael Matheson, MSP, Cabinet Secretary for NHS Recovery, Health and Social Care, regarding your experience of Queen Elizabeth University Hospital and your intention to publish a book.

Everyone who works in our Health Service must have the confidence to speak up and raise any concerns they may have. The Scottish Government expects all Health Boards and their staff to act according to NHS Scotland's values and behaviours.

When a whistleblower raises a concern, the Health Secretary stresses that this must be seriously and thoroughly investigated. It is imperative that the individual raising the concern does not suffer any repercussions for doing so. There are policies in place to support this, including the NHS Scotland Whistleblowing Policy (set against the National Whistleblowing Standards and Independent National Whistleblowing Officer role delivered by the Scottish Public Services Ombudsman); an independent advice line. To encourage and support staff in speaking up there is also a dedicated Whistleblowing Champions within each health board.

I hope this is of help and clarifies the position of the Scottish Government.

Yours sincerely

**** *****

**Workforce Practice** [1]

---

[1] This email has been paraphrased.

# Authors

**Yvonne Bennett**

I obtained my BA and MA through the Open University. On leaving school, I trained as a nurse and, after having my children, retrained as a nursery schoolteacher. I have completed a PhD at Canterbury Christ Church University. My research area of interest is conservative Presbyterianism in the Gàidhealtachd (Highlands and Islands) of Scotland. In 2021 I published a book which examines the ways in which churches in Britain help the vulnerable in their communities. The book *The Church Who Needs It? We Do!* examines the difficulties a group of South London women experience with Universal Credit and life under lockdown during the Coronavirus pandemic. In 2022, I edited a book, *Women and Religion in Britain Today Belonging* with Vernon Press.

**Christina Stead**

I studied History at Durham University and then worked as an academic administrator and manager for a university in London. After a period of working in an educational consultancy, I took a career break when my daughter was born in 2004. Seeking new challenges, I volunteered in my local community and then retrained as a careers counsellor, gaining an MA (Distinction) from Canterbury Christ Church University in 2014. I was then awarded a scholarship by the university to pursue doctoral research, and my PhD (2020) explored the career paths of senior professional women in accountancy, education and medicine. I am currently working as a mentor to a student who is completing a doctorate in Nursing, and I am a school governor with a brief that includes safeguarding.

# Reference List

Adams, S. and Bancroft, H. (2020) "Did care homes use powerful sedatives to speed Covid deaths? Number of prescriptions for the drug midazolam doubled during height of the pandemic." *Mail on Sunday*. Available at: https://www.dailymail.co.uk/news/article-8514081/Number-prescriptions-drug-midazolam-doubled-height-pandemic.html. Accessed: 1st September 2023.

Adjepong, A. (2017) 'Invading ethnography: A queer of color reflexive practice.' *Ethnography*, 2019, 20 (1) pp. 27-46.

Aitkin, V. (2023) "NHS whistleblower slams health board at infection scandal hospital over 'toxic culture'." The Daily Record. Available at: https://www.dailyrecord.co.uk/news/scottish-news/scots-health-board-boss-made-3014 4488#ICID=Android_DailyRecordNewsApp_AppShare. Accessed: 1st September 2023.

Age Concern (2023) *Fixing the foundations. Why it's time to rethink how we support older people with health problems to stay well at home.* Available at: age-uk-report---fixing-the-foundations-feb-2023.pdf (ageuk.org.uk). Accessed: 8th November 2023.

Alexander, S. (2013) "'As long as it helps somebody': why vulnerable people participate in research." *International Journal of Palliative Nursing*, volume 16(4), pp. 174 – 180. Available at: https://doi.org/10.12968/ijpn.2010.16.4.47 783. Accessed: 23rd October 2023.

Amarante, I. (2023) "Why the care industry needs greater gender diversity." *Halescare Homecare* Blog. Available at: https://halescare.co.uk/care-industry -needs-greater-gender-diversity/. Accessed: 20th October 2023.

Anderson, C., Grey, T., Kennelly, S. and O'Neill, D. (2020) "Nursing home design and COVID-19: balancing infection control, quality of life and resilience." *JAMADA*, volume 21, pp. 1519 -1524.

Anderson, H. (2023) "Government reveals new private hospital contract costs." Health and Care Scotland. Available at: https://healthandcare.scot/stories/ 2626/k/#:~:text=According%20to%20the%20Public%20Contracts,the%20final %20cost%20would%20higher. Accessed: 12th September 2023.

Andrews, A., Squire, C. and Tamboukou, M. (eds.) (2013) *Doing Narrative Research (2nd ed)*. London: Sage.

Andrews, M. (2013) "Never the last word: revisiting data", in Andrews, M., Squire, C. and Tamboukou, M. (eds.) *Doing Narrative Research*. London: Sage, pp. 205 - 222.

Andruske, C. L., and O'Connor, D. (2020) "Family care across diverse cultures: Re-envisioning using a transnational lens." *Journal of Aging Studies*, volume, 55, pp. 1 – 10.

Appleby, J. and Gainsbury S. (2022) The past, present and future government spending on the NHS. The Nutfield Trust. Available at: https://www.nuffield trust.org.uk/news-item/the-past-present-and-future-of-government-spending-on-the-nhs. Accessed: 2nd July 2023.

Ashrafi, S. R. H. N. (2017) *Ethical Principles for Hospital Design.* PhD Thesis, Liverpool, The University of Liverpool. Available at: https://livrepository.liverpool. ac.uk/3022732/. Accessed: 1st October 2023.

Association of Ambulance Chief Executives (2023) "Violence, aggression and abuse." Available at: https://aace.org.uk/vaa/#:~:text=Every%20day%20during% 20the%202020,over%20the%20last%20five%20years. Accessed: 4th November 2023.

Audit Scotland (2023) *The NHS in Scotland 2022.* Available at: https://www. audit-scotland.gov.uk/uploads/docs/report/2023/nr_230223_nhs_overview. pdf. Accessed: 20th July 2023.

Auth, N. M., Booker, M. J., Wild, J. and Riley, R., (2022) "Mental health and help seeking among trauma-exposed emergency service staff: a qualitative evidence synthesis." *BMJ Open.* Available at: https://bmjopen.bmj.com/content/12/ 2/e047814. Accessed: 1st September 2023.

Bambi, S., Foà, C., De Felippis, C., Lucchini, A., Guazzini, A. and Rasero, L. (2018). "Workplace incivility, lateral violence, and bullying among nurses. A review about their prevalence and related factors." *Acta Biomed,* volume 89 (6), pp. 51 – 79.

Ben-Harush, A., Shiovitz-Ezra, S., Doron, I., Alon., S., Leibovitz, A., Golander, H., Haron, Y. and Ayalon, L. (2017) "Ageism among physicians, nurses, and social workers: findings from a qualitative study." *EUR J Ageing,* volume 14, pp. 39 – 48.

Bennett, Y. H. (2020) *"Because the Bible Tells Me So": Gender and authority in conservative Presbyterianism on the Isle of Lewis (Scotland).* PhD Thesis, Canterbury, Canterbury Christ Church University.

Berry, W. (2021) "The psychology of complaining: With complaining being viewed so negatively, why is it so prevalent?" *Psychology Today.* Available at: https://www.psychologytoday.com/gb/blog/the-second-noble-truth/202104/ the-psychology-complaining. Accessed: 20th May 2024.

BJGP Life (2022) "Fining patients who miss GP appointments – will this strategy work?" Available at: https://bjgplife.com/fining-patients-who-miss-gp-appointments-will-this-strategy-work/. Accessed: 10th November 2023.

Blumer, H. (1969) *Symbolic Interactionism: Perspective and Method.* London: The University of California Press.

BMA (2022) "The country is getting sicker: The urgent need to address growing health inequalities and protect our health in the face of an economic crisis." Available at: https://trfthealthweeklydigest.wordpress.com/2022/12/19/the-country-is-getting-sicker-the-urgent-need-to-address-growing-health-inequalities-and-protect-our-health-in-the-face-of-an-economic-crisis/. Accessed: 10th July 2023.

Booth, R. and Goodier, M. (2023) "Number of adults living with parents in England and Wales rises by 700,000 in a decade." The Guardian, 10th May 2023. Available at: https://www.theguardian.com/society/2023/may/10/number -adults-living-parents-england-wales-up-700000-decade. Accessed: 21st July 2024.

Bows, H. and Herring, J. (2022) "DNA/CPR Decisions During COVID – 19: An empirical and analytical study." *Medical Law Review,* volume 30(1), pp. 60 – 80.

Bugelli, V., Campobasso, C. P., Feola, A., Abbruzzese, A. and Di Paolo, M. (2023) "Accidental injury or 'shaken elderly syndrome'? Insights from a case report. *Healthcare*, volume 11(2) p. 228. Available at: https://www.mdpi.com/2227-9032/11/2/228. Accessed: 10th May 2024.

Burkitt, R., Duxbury, K., Evans, H., Ewbank, L., Gregory, F., Hall, S,, Wellings, D. and Wenzel L. (2018) *The public and the NHS: what's the deal?* London: The King's Fund. Available at: www.kingsfund. org.uk/publications/public-and-nhs-whats-the-deal. Accessed 10th May 2024.

Campbell D. (2022) "More than half of NHS paramedics suffering from burnout, study finds." *The Guardian*, 6th February 2022. Available at: https://www.theguardian.com/society/2022/feb/06/more-than-half-of-nhs-paramedics-suffering-from-burnout-study-finds#:~:text=Over%20half%20of%20paramedics%20are,service%2C%20a%20study%20has%20found. Accessed 1st September 2023.

Care Information Scotland (2023) "Personal and nursing care in homes." Available at: https://careinfoscotland.scot/topics/care-homes/paying-care-home-fees/personal-and-nursing-care-in-care-homes/. Accessed: 31st October 2023.

Carvalho dos Santos, J. and Ceolim, M. F. (2007) "Nursing iatrogenic events in hospitalised elderly patients." *Revista da Escola de Enfermagem da USP,* volume 43(4), pp. 810-817. Available at: https://www.scielo.br/j/reeusp/a/qQxM8PdXSZCBnWXGskBNBSm/?lang=en. Accessed: 20th August 2023.

Chang, H. (2008) *Autoethnography as a Method.* London: Routledge Taylor Francis.

Cherniack, E. P. (2002) "Increasing use of DNR orders in the elderly worldwide: whose choice is it?" *J Med Ethics*, volume 28(5), pp. 303 – 307. Available at: https://www.ncbi.nlm.nih.gov/pmc/articles/PMC1733661/. Accessed: October 1st 2023.

Church, E. (2023) "Student nurse demand improvements to bursary as many consider dropping out." *Nursing Times*. Available at: https://www.nursingtimes.net/news/education/student-nurses-demand-improvements-to-bursary-as-many-consider-dropping-out-28-06-2023/#:~:text=Almost%20all%20(98%25)%20of,to%20£10%2C000%20in%202021.Accessed: 10th May 2024.

Cierelli, V. G. (1981) *Helping Elderly Parents: The Role of Adult Children.* Boston: Auburn House Publishing Company.

Cohen, S. (2020) *The NHS: Britain's National Health Service, 1948 – 2020.* Glasgow: Bell and Bain Ltd.

Coleman, V. (2022) *NHS: What's Wrong and How to Put it Right.* Great Britain: Amazon.

Connell, R. W. and Messerschmidt, J. W. (2005) "Hegemonic Masculinity: Rethinking the Concept." *Gender and Society*, volume 19(6), pp. 829-859.

Cummings, B. (2023) "Pig Iron: *The Kaleidoscope. Tortoise Investigations* (4). Available at: https://www.tortoisemedia.com/audio/pig-iron-the-kaleidoscope/. Accessed: 24th September 2023. Denzin, N., and Lincoln, Y. (2011b) "The discipline and practice of qualitative research." Denzin, N. and Lincoln, Y. (eds) *The Sage Handbook of Qualitative Research, (4th ed)*. Thousand Oaks, CA: Sage, pp. 1 - 20.

Department of Health and Social Care (2015) *The NHS Constitution for England.* Available at: https://www.gov.uk/government/publications/the-nhs-constitution-for-england/the-nhs-constitution-for-england. Accessed: 1st October 2023.

Devereux, E. (2023) "Nurse retention plan urgently needed, Scottish Government warned." *Nursing Times*, 3rd May 2023. Available at: https://www.nursing times.net/news/workforce/nurse-retention-plan-urgently-needed-scottish-government-warned-03-05-2023/. Accessed: 10th May 2024.

Ellis, P. and Standing, M. (2023*) Patient Assessment and Care Planning in Nursing.* London: Learning Matters, A SAGE Publishing Company.

Elston, J., Gradinger, F., Asthana, S., Lilley-Woolnough, C., Wroe, S., Harman, H., and Byng, R. (2019) "Does a social prescribing 'holistic' link-worker for older people with complex, multimorbidity improve well-being and frailty and reduce health and social care use and costs? A 12 month before-and-after evaluation." *Primary Health Care Research and Development*, volume 20(e135), pp.1 - 10. Cambridge: Cambridge University Press.

Etherington, K. (2004) *Becoming a Reflexive Researcher: Using Our Selves in Research.* London: Jessica Kingsley.

Fetzer, T. (2019) "Did Austerity Cause Brexit?" *American Economic Review,* volume 109 (11), pp. 3849 – 86. Available at: https://www.aeaweb.org/articles?id=10. 1257/aer.20181164. Accessed: 21st July 2024.

Finch, D., Wilson, H. and Bibby, J. (2023) "Leave no one behind: The State of health and health inequalities in Scotland." The Health Foundation. Available at: https://www.health.org.uk/sites/default/files/upload/publications/2023/HF_ Health_Scotland_Web_Final.pdf. Accessed: 21st July 2024.

Fivush, R. (2019). "Family narratives and the development of an autobiographical self: Social and cultural perspectives on autobiographical memory." APA PsycNet. Available at: https://psycnet.apa.org/record/2019-13704-000. Accessed: 21st June 2024.

Gilmore, K., J., Corazza, I., Coletta, L. and Allin, S. (2023) "The uses of patient reported experience measures in health systems: a systemic narrative review." *Health Policy*, volume 128, pp. 1 – 10. Available at: https://www.sciencedirect. com/science/article/pii/S0168851022001920. Accessed: 8th May 2024.

Goffman, E. (1963) *Stigma: Notes on the Management of Spoiled Identity.* New Jersey: Prentice Hall.

Goffman, E. (1959) *The Presentation of Self in Everyday Life.* London: Penguin.

Gordon, T. (2020) "Angus Robertson slated for saying elderly deaths a 'gain' for independence amid pandemic." *The Herald*, 20th September 2020. Available at: https://www.heraldscotland.com/news/18734202.angus-robertson-slated -saying-elderly-deaths-gain-independence-amid-pandemic/. Accessed: 1st September 2023.

Green, D., Filkin, G. and Woods, T. (2021) "Our unhealthy nation." The Lancet, volume 2(1) pp. 8-9. Available at: https://www.thelancet.com/journals/lanhl/ article/PIIS2666-7568(20)30062-3/fulltext. Accessed: 20th September 2023.8

Hall, R. (2022) "What are the NHS ambulance response categories?" *The Guardian,* 20th December 2022. Available at: https://www.theguardian.com/society/ 2022/dec/20/what-are-the-nhs-ambulance-response-categories. Accessed 7th November 2023.

Halpern, J., Gurevich, M., Schwartz, B. and Brazaeu, P. (2009) "Interventions for critical incident stress in emergency medical services: a qualitative study." *Stress and Health*, volume 25(2), pp. 139 – 149.

Hammett, E. (2023) "999 – when to call for an ambulance and when not to." *First Aid for Life*. Available at: https://firstaidforlife.org.uk/999when-to-call-for-an-ambulance-and-when-not-to/. Accessed: 7th November 2023.

Haraway, D. (1988) "Situated knowledges: the science question in feminism and the privilege of partial perspective." *Feminist Studies*, volume 14(3), pp. 575 – 99.

Health Improvement Scotland (2019) *Unannounced Inspection Report – Safety and Cleanliness of Hospitals Queen Elizabeth University Hospital (including Institute of Neurosciences and Royal Hospital for Children) NHS Greater Glasgow and Clyde 29–31 January 2019*. Available at: https://archive2021.parliament.scot/S5_HealthandSportCommittee/Inquiries/20190308_QEUH_safety_and_cleanliness_inspection_report.pdf. Accessed: 14th November 2023.

Healthcare Improvement Scotland (2024) "What does Healthcare Improvement Scotland do when a concern is raised." *Healthcare Improvement Scotland*. Available at: https://www.healthcareimprovementscotland.scot/improving-care/responding-to-concerns/what-does-healthcare-improvement-scotland-do-when-a-concern-is-received/. Accessed 20th May 2024.

Hervieu Léger, D. (2000) *Religion as a Chain of Memory*. Cambridge: Polity Press.

HESA (2021) *Figure 11 - Standard industrial classification of graduates entering work in the UK by subject area of degree*. Available at: https://www.hesa.ac.uk/data-and-analysis/sb266/figure-11 Accessed: 10th May 2024.

Hodkinson, P. and Hodkinson, H. (2001) "The strengths and limitations of case study research." *Making an Impact on Policy and Practice Conference*, Learning and Skills Development Agency, Cambridge, 5 - 7 December.

Hollway, W. and Jefferson, T. (2013) *Doing Qualitative Research Differently: A Psychosocial Approach (2nd ed)*. London: Sage Publications.

Holroyd-Leduc, J., Resin, J., Ashley, L., Barwich, D., Elliott, J., Huras, P., Légaré F., Mahoney, M., Matbee, A., McNeil, H., Pullman, D., Sawatzky, R. and Stolee, P. (2016) "Giving voice to older adults living with frailty and their family caregivers: engagement of older adults living with frailty in research, health care decision making, and in health policy." *Research, Involvement and Engagement*, volume 2(23), pp. 1 – 19.

Horsdal, M. (2012) *Telling lives. Exploring dimensions of narratives*. Abingdon: Routledge. Huffington, A. (2015) "What's working: all the news that's fit to print." *Huffington Post* Available at: https://www.huffpost.com/entry/whats-working-all-the-news_b_6603924. Accessed: 12th September 2023.

Indeed Careers Guide (2023) "What is the importance of knowing your team? (With Benefits)." Available at: https://uk.indeed.com/career-advice/career-development/knowing-your-team#:~:text=It%20improves%20workplace%20productivity,position%20to%20create%20these%20environments. Accessed: 12th November 2023.

Jackson, J. (2023) *"Becoming the midwife I have in my head': A qualitative multiple case study of midwifery students."* PhD Thesis, Canterbury, Canterbury Christ Church University. Available at: https://repository.canterbury.ac.uk/download/239d0a8ff760f15bd49be1b4326b73f6f6a4c4fb521bd7d3299839da338fd923/5849075/Judith%20Jackson%20NAB%2091999329%20Final%20Thesis.pdf Accessed: 27th May 2024.

Jeffries, D., Wellings, D., Morris, J., Dayan, M. and Lobont, C. (2023) "Public satisfaction with the NHS and social care in 2023: Results from the British Social Attitudes Survey." Nuffield Trust. Available at: https://www.nuffieldtrust. org.uk/sites/default/files/2024-03/BSA%20Survey%202023_FINAL.pdf. Accessed: 21st July 2024.

Johansson, F. (2004) *The Medici Effect: Breakthrough Insights at the Intersection of Ideas, Concepts and Cultures*. Boston: Harvard Business School Press.

Johnson, S. (2023) "Scotland's largest health board a formal suspect in corporate homicide investigation." *The Telegraph*. Available at: https://www.telegraph. co.uk/news/2023/11/12/scotland-health-board-suspect-corporate-homicide -probe/. Accessed: 14th November 2023.

Jones, J. (2020) *Can You Hear Me?* London: Quercus.

Josselson, R. (2009) "The present of the past. Dialogues with memory over time." *Journal of Personality*, volume 77(3), pp. 647 - 668.

Katz-Rothman, B. (2007) "Writing Ourselves in Sociology." *Methodological Innovations Online*, volume 2(1), pp.11 - 16.

Kelly, L. A., Faan, R. N., Gee, P. M. and Butler, R. J. (2021) "Impact of nurse burnout on organizational and position turnover." *Nursing Outlook*, volume 69(1), pp. 96 - 102. Available at: https://pubmed.ncbi.nlm.nih.gov/33023759/. Accessed: 12th September 2023.

Khraief, C., Benzarti, F. and Amiri, H. (2020) "Elderly fall detection based on multi-stream deep convolutional networks." *Multimed Tools Appl*, volume 79, pp. 19537 – 19560. Available at: https://link.springer.com/article/10.1007/ s11042-020-08812-x. Accessed 10th May 2024.

Koch, T. (1990) Mirrored Lives: *Aging Children and Elderly Parents*. New York: Praeger Publishers.

Leask, D. (2016) "Queen Elizabeth University Hospital under fire over suicides." *The Herald* Available at: https://www.heraldscotland.com/news/14594183. queen-elizabeth-university-hospital-fire-suicides/. Accessed: 10th November 2023.

Leigh Day (2014) *Landmark judgement in resuscitation case*. London: Leigh Day Law Firm, Available at: https://www.leighday.co.uk/news/news/2014- news/landmark-judgment-in-resuscitation-case/#:~:text=The%20Court%20 of%20Appeal%20in,placed%20on%20her%20medical%20records. Accessed: August 30th 2023.

Leys, C. (2020) "How a decade of Austerity Brought the NHS to its Knees." *Tribune*, Available at: https://tribunemag.co.uk/2020/07/how-a-decade-of- austerity-brought-the-nhs-to-its-knees. Accessed: 10th November 2023.

Leith, M. S. and Sim, D. (2022) "'Will ye no' comeback again?': population challenge and diaspora policy in Scotland." *Population, Space and Place*, volume 28, pp. 1 – 10. Available at: https://doi.org/10.1002/psp.2572. Accessed: June 30th 2023.

Lothian, K. and Philp, I. (2001) "Care of older people: maintaining the dignity and autonomy of older people in the healthcare setting." *BMJ*, volume 322, pp. 688 – 670.

Lutova, L., Karisalmi, N., Aarikka-Stenroos, L. and Kaipio, J. (2019) "Comparing three methods to capture multidimensional service experience in children's health care: video diaries, narratives, and semi structured interviews."

*International Journal of Qualitative Methods*, volume 18, pp. 1 – 13. Available at: https://journals.sagepub.com/doi/epub/10.1177/1609406919835112. Accessed: 1st September 2023.

Macgill, J. and Pringle, E. (2023) "NHS boards' 'unprecedented' budget challenges.", 8th November 2023. Available at: https://healthandcare.scot/stories/3368/k/ Accessed: 11th November 2023. McArdle, H. (2024) "Glasgow superhospital: HIS apology over probe 'shortcomings'." *The Herald*. Available at: https://www.heraldscotland.com/news/24208205.glasgow-superhospital-apology-probe-shortcomings/. Accessed: 20th May 2024.

McCarthy, C. S. (2020) *Traditional Emergency Department or Emergency Nurse Led Minor Injury Unit: Predicting Patient Choice for Delivery of Minor Injury Care*. PhD Thesis, School of Healthcare Studies, Cardiff University.

McCartney, G., McMaster, R., Popham, F., Dundas, R. and Walsh, D. (2022) "Is austerity a cause of slower improvements in mortality in high-income countries? A panel analysis." *Social Science and Medicine*, volume, 313. Available at: https://www.sciencedirect.com/science/article/pii/S0277953622007031. Accessed: 24th July 2024.

McCrone, D. (2017) *The New Sociology of Scotland*. London: SAGE Publications.

McGill, S. and Duffy, A. (2022) "Glasgow great-gran endured five hours 'screaming in agony' on care home floor waiting on ambulance." *Glasgow Live*. Available at: https://www.glasgowlive.co.uk/news/glasgow-news/glasgow-great-gran-endured-five-24758473. Accessed: 1st September 2023.

McKee, M., Dunnell, K., Anderson, M., Brayne, C. and Charlesworth, A. (2021) "The changing health needs of the UK population." *The Lancet*. volume 397, pp. 1979 – 1991.

McLardy-Smith, P. (2022) *Eden is Burning: What next for the NHS*. London: Bite Sized Books.

McMahon, C. (2019) *The Psychology of Social Media*. London: Routledge.

McQueenie, R., Ellis, A., McConnachie, A., Wilson, P. and Williamson, A. E. (2019) "Morbidity, mortality and missed appointments in healthcare: a national retrospective data linkage study." BMC Medicine, volume 17(2) pp. 1 – 8. Available at: https://bmcmedicine.biomedcentral.com/articles/10.1186/s12916-018-1234-0. Accessed: 10th November 2023.

Mapedzahama, V. and Dune T. (2017) A Clash of Paradigms? *Ethnography and Ethics Approval* Sage Open, Jan-March 2017: pp. 1-8.

Mars, B., Hird, K., Bell, F., James, C. and Gunnell, D. (2020) "Suicide among ambulance service staff: a review of coroner and employment records." *British Paramedic Journal*, volume 4(4), pp. 10 – 15.

Mavin, S., Grandyland, G. and Williams, J. (2014) "Experiences of women elite leaders doing gender: intra-gender micro-violence between women." *British Journal of Management*, volume 25, pp. 439 – 455.

Maines, M. J, Pierce, J. L. and Laslett, B. (2008) *Telling Stories: The use of personal narrative in the social sciences and history*. New York: Cornell University.

Mendes, P. N., do Livramento Fortes Figueiredo, M., Ribeiro dos Santos, A. M., Fernandes, M. A. and Fonseca, R., S., B. (2018) "Physical, emotional and social burden of elderly parents 'informal caregivers." *Acta Paul Enferm*, volume 32(1), pp. 87 – 94.

Merrill, B. and West, L. (2009) *Using Biographical Methods in Social Research.* London: Sage.

Mitchell, G. (2021) "Clap for heroes: nurses say they do not want return of applause. *Nursing Times,* 07 January 2021. Available at: Clap for Heroes: Nurses say they do not want return of applause | Nursing Times. Accessed: 9th November 2023.

Morgan, D. L. and Guevera, H. (2008) "Rapport" in Given, L. M (ed) *The SAGE Encyclopedia of Qualitative Research Methods.* Thousand Oaks: Sage Publications.

National Records of Scotland (2022) *Healthy Life Expectancy 2018 - 2020.* Available at: https://www.nrscotland.gov.uk/files/statistics/healthy-life-expectancy/18-20/healthy-life-expectancy-18-20-report.pdf. Accessed: 20th August 2023.

National Records of Scotland (2023) *Life Expectancy in Scotland 2019-2021.* Available at: https://www.nrscotland.gov.uk/files/statistics/life-expectancy-in-scotland/19-21/life-expectancy-19-21-report.pdf. Accessed: 20th August 2023.

Neimeyer, R. A. and Stewart, A. E. (1996) "Trauma, healing, and the narrative employment of loss." *Families in Society: The Journal of Contemporary Human Services*, volume 77(6) pp. 360 – 375.

NHS Digital (2023) *NHS Sickness Absence Days, March 2023.* Available at: https://journals.sagepub.com/doi/10.1606/1044-3894.933. Accessed: 11th October 2023.

NHS England (2019) *Missed GP appointments costing NHS millions.* Available at: https://www.england.nhs.uk/2019/01/missed-gp-appointments-costing-nhs-millions/. Accessed: 10th November 2023.

NHS England (2020) "Retention Interventions Examples." Available at: https://www.england.nhs.uk/looking-after-our-people/supporting-people-in-early-and-late-career/retention-interventions-examples/. Accessed: 10th May 2024.

NHS Research Authority (2023) "Communicating study findings to participants: guidance." *NHS Research Authority.* Available at: Communicating study findings to participants: guidance - Health Research Authority (hra.nhs.uk). Accessed: 24th October 2023.

NHS Scotland (2022) *NHS Scotland performance against LDP standards.* Available at: https://www.gov.scot/publications/nhsscotland-performance-against-ldp-standards/pages/sickness-absence/. Accessed: 11th October 2023.

NHS Scotland (2021) *Whislteblowing Policy. Workforce Policies.* Available at: https://workforce.nhs.scot/policies/whistleblowing-policy/. Accessed: 10th October 2023.

Northumbria University (2023) *Nursing science registered nurse (adult) BSc (hons)* Available at: Adult Nursing Degree BSc (Hons) | Adult Nurse Course | Northumbria. Accessed: 1st November 2023.

Nurses.co.uk (2023) "Stats and facts on the UK's nursing workforce 2023." Available at: Stats And Facts On The UK's Nursing Workforce 2023 (nurses.co.uk). Accessed 30th October 2023.

Nursing and Midwifery Council (2023) Leavers' survey 2022. Available at: https://www.nmc.org.uk/news/news-and-updates/record-number-of-nurses-midwives-and-nursing-associates/. Accessed: 10th April 2024.

Nursing and Midwifery Council (2018) "The code: professional standards of practice and behaviour for nurses, midwives and nursing associates." Available at: https://www.nmc.org.uk/globalassets/sitedocuments/nmc-publications/nmc-code.pdf. Accessed: 3rd November 2023.

Oakley, A. (1981) "Interviewing women: a contradiction in terms." Roberts, H. (ed.) *Doing Feminist Research*. London: Kegan Paul, pp. 30 - 61.

Office for National Statistics (2022) "Health state life expectancies, UK: 2018-2021". Available at: https://www.ons.gov.uk/peoplepopulationandcommunity/healthandsocialcare/healthandlifeexpectancies/bulletins/healthstatelifeexpectanciesuk/2018to2020. Accessed: 20th August 2023.

Page, R. (2018) *Narratives Online: Shared Stories in Social Media*. Cambridge: Cambridge University Press.

Parker, K. J., Phiilips, J. L., Luckett, T., Agar, M., Ferguson, C. and Hickmann, L. D. (2021) "Analysis of discharge documentation for older adults living with dementia: A cohort study". *Journal of Clinical Nursing*, volume 31, pp. 13 – 14. Available at: https://onlinelibrary.wiley.com/doi/abs/10.1111/jocn.15885. Accessed 10th May 2024.

Parliamentary and Health Service Ombudsman (2015) *Breaking down the barriers: Older people and their complaints about health care*. Available at: https://www.ombudsman.org.uk/sites/default/files/Breaking_down_the_barriers_report.pdf. Accessed: 14th November 2023.

Parry, H. (2015) "Nicola's Death Star strikes back: now visitors to £1billion Glasgow super-hospital get stuck in the lifts…. Because they have no buttons inside." *Mailonline*. Available at: https://www.dailymail.co.uk/news/article-3075600/Visitors-1billion-super-hospital-getting-stuck-lifts-no-buttons-inside.html#:~:text=The%20issue%20arises%20from%20the,how%20to%20use%20them%20properly. Accessed: 1st October 2023.

Pascoe Leahy, C. (2022) "The afterlife of interviews: explicit ethics and subtle ethics in sensitive or distressing qualitative research." *Qualitative Research*, volume 22(5), pp. 777 - 794. Available at: https://doi.org/10.1177/1468794121 1012924. Accessed: 23rd October 2023.

Peavy, R. (1992) "A constructivist model of training for career counsellors." *Journal of Career Development*, volume 18(3), pp. 215 - 28.

Permpongkosol, S. (2011) "Iatrogenic disease in the elderly: risk factors, consequences, and prevention." *Clinical Interventions in Aging*. 2011(6) pp. 77 - 82.

Phoenix, A. (2013) "Analysing narrative contexts.", in Andrews, M. Squire C. and Tambouko, M. (eds) *Doing Narrative Research*, pp. 72 – 87. London: Sage.

Pilnick, A. (2023) "What's wrong with patient centred care? A sociological critique." *Everyday Society. The British Sociological Association*, 24th October 2023, pp. 1 – 7. Available at: https://es.britsoc.co.uk/whats-wrong-with-patient-centred-care-a-sociological-critique/. Accessed: 31st October 2023.

Plummer, K. (2001) *Documents of Life 2: An Invitation to a Critical Humanism*. London: Sage.

Public Health Scotland (2023) *Delayed discharges in NHS Scotland, annual: Annual summary of occupied beds and census figures, data to March 2023. Edinburgh*: A National Statistics publication for Scotland. Available at: https://publichealthscotland.scot/publications/delayed-discharges-in-nhsscotland-annual/delayed-discharges-in-nhsscotland-annual-annual-summary-of-occupied-bed-days-and-census-figures-data-to-march-2023/. Accessed: 10th October 2023.

Putnam, L. L. and Banghart, S. (2017) "Interpretive Approaches' The International Encyclopaedia of Organisational Communication." Available at: https://online library.wiley.com/doi/abs/10.1002/9781118955567.wbieoc118 Accessed: 24th July 2024.

Quallington, J. (2015) "The nursing shortfall is a ticking time bomb." *Health Services Journal.* Available at: The nursing shortfall is a ticking time bomb | Comment | Health Service Journal (hsj.co.uk). Accessed: 7th November 2023.

Richardson, L. (1997) *Fields of Play: Constructing an Academic Life.* New Brunswick, N. J.: Rutgers University Press.

Riessman, C. (2008) *Narrative methods for the human sciences.* Thousand Oaks C. A.: Sage.

Riley, R. and Causer, H. (2023) "Why do NHS staff need suicide postvention?" *National Health Executive,* Sept/Oct 2023, pp. 36 - 37. Available at: https://mag.nationalhealthexecutive.com/articles/why-do-nhs-staff-need-suicide-postvention-?m=62920&i=801866&view=articleBrowser&article_id=4641371&ver=html5. Accessed: 12th September 2023.

Ris, I., Schnepp, W. and Imhof, R. M. (2018) "An integrative review on family caregivers 'involvement in care of home dwelling elderly." *Health and Social Care Community,* volume 27, pp. 95 – 111. Available at: https://pubmed.ncbi.nlm.nih.gov/30307685/. Accessed: 30th October 2023.

Robertson, C. and Rodgers, H. (2023) "Toxic dust from demolition site contaminated water supply at Glasgow's QEUH leading to killer infections." Daily Record. Available at: https://www.dailyrecord.co.uk/news/scottish-news/toxic-dust-demolition-site-contaminated-30032386#ICID=Android_DailyRecordNews App_AppShare. Accessed: June 30th 2023.

Royal College of Nursing (Scotland), (2023) *Nursing student finance: the true cost of becoming a nurse.* London: Royal College of Nursing

Royal College of Nursing (Scotland) (2022) *Nursing Under Pressures: Staffing for safe and effective care in Scotland.* London: Royal College of Nursing.

Sampath, R. (2022) "When is Iatrogenic Harm Negligent" *AMA Journal of Ethics,* volume 24(8), pp. 735 -739.

Savickas, M. (2011) *Career Counselling.* Washington DC.: American Psychological Association.

Scheff, T. J. (2003) "Shame in Self and Society." *Symbolic Interaction,* volume 26(2) pp. 239-262.

Scottish Government (2018) *Every life matters – Scotland's suicide prevention action plan.* Edinburgh: Scottish Government.

Scottish Government (2021) *A Scotland for the future: opportunities and challenges of Scotland's changing population.* Available at: https://www.gov.scot/publications/scotland-future-opportunities-challenges-scotlands-changing-population. Accessed 23rd September 2023.

Scottish Government (2021) *Healthy Living: Increasing Healthy Life Expectancy And Driving Innovation In An Ageing Society.* Available at: https://www.gov.scot/publications/scotland-future-opportunities-challenges-scotlands-changing-population/pages/6/. Accessed: 6th June 2023.

Scottish Government (2022) *Charter of patient rights and responsibilities – revised: June 2022.* Available at: https://www.gov.scot/publications/charter-patient-rights-responsibilities-revised-june-2022/. Accessed: 1st November 2023.

Scottish Government (2022) *Free Personal and Social Nursing Care, Scotland, 2020 – 2021.* Available at: https://www.gov.scot/publications/free-personal-nursing-care-scotland-2020-21/pages/3/. Accessed: 31st October 2023.

Scottish Government (2023) *Patient Safety Commissioner Bill passed.* Available at: https://www.gov.scot/news/patient-safety-commissioner-bill-passed/. Accessed 14th May 2024.

Scottish Hospital Inquiries (2023) *Provisional Position Paper 5 The History of Infection Concerns (HOIC) for the Queen Elizabeth University Hospital Campus.* Available at: https://www.hospitalsinquiry.scot/inquiry-document/history-infection-concerns-hoic-queen-elizabeth-university-hospital-campus Accessed: 13th November 2023.

Scottish Labour (2021) *QEUH scandal: a timeline summary.* Available at: https://scottishlabour.org.uk/blog/qeuhtimeline/. Accessed: 11th November 2023.

Scottish National Party (2022) *Mitigating their mistakes: here's how the SNP is delivering for Scotland.* Available at: Mitigating their mistakes: Here's how the SNP is delivering for Scotland — Scottish National Party. Accessed: 31st October 2023.

Scott, J. (2019) "What are emergency ambulance services doing to meet the needs of people who call frequently? A national survey of current practice in the United Kingdom." *BMC, Emergency Medicine,* volume 19(82), pp. 1 – 8.

Selman, L. E., Sowden, R. and Borgstrom, E. (2021). "Saying 'goodbye' during the COVID-19 pandemic: A document analysis of online newspapers with implications for end-of-life care." *Palliative Medicine,* volume 35(7), pp. 1277 - 1287. Available at: https://doi.org/10.1177/02692163211017023. Accessed: 21st June 2024.

Sheppard, L. D. and Aquino, K. (2017) 'Sisters at Arms: A Theory of Female Same-Sex Conflict and It's Problematization in Organizations'. *Journal of Management,* volume 43(3) pp.691-715.

Sherrell, K. and Newton, N. (1996) "Parent Care as a Developmental Task." *Families in Society: The Journal of Contemporary Human Services,* volume 77(3) pp. 174 – 181.

Shi, Y. (2021) *First-Person Narrative and Story Meaningfulness: Promoting Empathy via Storytelling.* A paper submitted in partial fulfilment of the requirements for the Master of Arts degree in the Master of Arts Program in the Social Sciences, The University of Chicago.

Shibutani, T. (1970) *Human Nature and Collective Behaviour: Papers in honour of Herbert Blumer.* Englewood Cliffs New Jersey: Prentice-Hall.

Shorey, S. and Wong, P., Z., E. (2021) "A qualitative systematic review on nurses' experiences of workplace bullying and implications for nursing practice." *Journal of Advanced Nursing,* volume 77(11), pp. 4291 – 4598.

Shutterstock (2024) Photograph of the Queen Elizabeth University Hospital, Glasgow. Purchased 30th July 2024. Available at: www.shutterstock.com. Accessed: 30th July 2024.

Singh, I. and Okeke, J. (2016) "Reducing inpatient falls in a 100% single room elderly care environment: evaluation of the impact of a systematic nurse training programme on falls risk assessment (FRA)." *BMJ Open Quality*, volume 5, pp 1 – 9. Available at: https://bmjopenquality.bmj.com/content/5/1/u210921.w4741.citation-tools. Accessed: 10th September 2023.

Sirrs, C. (2024) "The moment of patient safety: iatrogenic injury, clinical error and cultures of healthcare in the NHS." *Social History of Medicine*, volume 20, pp. 1 – 23. Available at: https://academic.oup.com/shm/advance-article/doi/10.1093/shm/hkad089/7627372. Accessed: 8th May 2024.

Smith, R. (2023) "Spending ever more on the NHS and less on education: is this sensible?" *BMJ*, volume 381, pp. 916-918. Available at: https://www.bmj.com/content/381/bmj.p916. Accessed: 1st September 2023.

Snooks, H. A., Khanom, A., Cole, R., Edwards, A., Mair Edwards, B., Evans, B. A., Foster, T., Fothergill, R. T., Gripper, C. P., Hampton, C. John, A., Petterson, R., Porter, A., Rosser, A. and Scott, J. (2019) "What are emergency ambulance services doing to meet the needs of people who call frequently? A national survey of current practice in the United Kingdom." *BMC Emergency Medicine*. Available at: https://bmcemergmed.biomedcentral.com/articles/10.1186/s1 2873-019-0297-3. Accessed: 10th October 2023.

Speedy, J. (2008) *Narrative Inquiry in Psychotherapy*. Basingstoke: Palgrave Macmillan.

Squire, C. (2013) "Experienced-centred and culturally-orientated approaches to narrative." In Andrews, M., Squire, C. and Tambouko, M. (eds) *Doing Narrative Research, (2nd ed)*, pp. 47-71. London: Sage.

Stanley, L. (1993) "On Auto/Biography in Sociology." *Sociology*, volume 27(1) pp. 41-52.

Stead, C. (2020) *Women at the School Gates: A Narrative Study of the Career Paths of Three Women*. PhD Thesis, Canterbury, Canterbury Christ Church University.

Stewart, E. A. (2023) *How Britain Loves the NHS*. Bristol: Policy Press. Available at: https://pureportal.strath.ac.uk/en/publications/how-britain-loves-the-nhs-practices-of-care-and-contestation. Accessed 10th May 2024.

Stuckler, D., Reeves, A., Loopstra, R., Karanikolos, M. and McKee, M. (2017) "Austerity and health: the impact in the UK and Europe." *European Journal of Public Health*, volume 27(4), pp.18 - 21. Available at: https://academic.oup.com/eurpub/article/27/suppl_4/18/4430523?login=false. Accessed: 3rd November 2023.

Taylor, S. (2011) "Why do the elderly allow the NHS to treat them so badly?" *The Guardian:* The Observer, GP. Available at: https://www.theguardian.com/commentisfree/2011/feb/20/elderly-need-specialist-doctors. Accessed: 12th July 2023.

Sutherland, R. (2018) "Tackling the root causes of suicide." NHS England: Blog. Available at: https://www.england.nhs.uk/blog/tackling-the-root-causes-of-suicide/. Accessed: 21st July 2024.

The Glasgow Indicators Project (2023) *Understanding Glasgow*. Available at: https://www.understandingglasgow.com. Accessed: 21st July 2024.

The Royal College of Nursing (2023) *Valuing Nursing in the UK: Staffing for safe and effective care in the UK, interventions to mitigate risks to nursing retention*. London: The Royal College of Nursing.

Tillman, L. (2015) *In Solidarity. Friendship, family and activism beyond gay and straight.* New York: Routledge.

Tomkow, L., Dewhurst, F., Hubmann, M., Straub, C., Damisa, E., Hanratty, B. and Todd, C. (2023) "'That's as hard a decision as you will ever have to make': the experiences of people who have discussed Do Not Attempt Cardiopulmonary Resuscitation on behalf of a relative during the COVID – 19 pandemic." *Age and Aging*, volume 52, pp. 1 – 9.

University of Hertfordshire (2023) *Health, nursing, midwifery and social work* Available at: Health, nursing, midwifery and social work | Courses | Uni of Herts. Accessed: 1st November 2023.

University of the West of Scotland (2023) *Adult nursing* Available at: BSc Adult Nursing | UWS | University of the West of Scotland. Accessed: 1st November.

Walsh D., McCartney G., Minton J., Parkinson, J., Shipton, D. and Whyte, B. (2021) Deaths from 'diseases of despair 'in Britain: comparing suicide, alcohol-related and drug-related mortality for birth cohorts in Scotland, England and Wales, and selected cities." *Journal of Epidemiology and Community Health*, volume 75, pp. 1195-1201.

Ward, S. and Brady, J. (2022) "Two patients' deaths blamed on staffing issues at the Queen Elizabeth University Hospital." *Daily Record*, 7th November 2022. Available at: https://www.dailyrecord.co.uk/news/scottish-news/two-patients-deaths-blamed-staffing-28426002. Accessed: 24th September 2023.

Webber, A. (2024) "Call for continued investment in NHS staff mental health hubs." *Occupational Health and Wellbeing Plus*, 27th March 2024. Available at: https://www.personneltoday.com/hr/nhs-mental-health-hubs-2024-investment/. Accessed: 27th May 2024.

West, L. (1996) *Beyond fragments. Adults, motivation and higher education. A biographical analysis.* London: Taylor and Francis.

Wilkinson, R. and Marmot, M. (eds) (2003) "The solid facts – the social determinants of health." *World Health Organisation.* Available at: EN: Social determinants of health. The solid facts (who.int). Accessed: 3rd November 2023.

Wright Mills, C. (1959) *The Sociological Imagination. Fortieth Edition.* Oxford: Oxford University Press.

Wyper, G. M. A., Mackay, D. F., Fraser, C., Lewsey, J., Robinson, M., Beeston, C. and Giles, L. (2023) "Evaluating the impact of alcohol minimum unit pricing on deaths and hospitalisations in Scotland: a controlled interrupted time series study." *The Lancet*, volume 401, pp. 1361 –1370.

Zazzara, M. B., Palmer, K., Vetrano, D. L., Carfi, A. and Onder, G. (2021) Adverse drug reactions in older adults: a narrative review of the literature. *European Geriatric Medicine*, volume 12, pp. 463 – 473. Available at: https://link.springer.com/article/10.1007/s41999-021-00481-9. Accessed: 10th May 2024.

# Index

# T

trauma: xi, xxiv, 6, 7, 20, 22-24, 26,
    28, 35, 42, 45, 46, 51, 52, 68, 75,
    107, 108, 118, 124

# V

voice: xi, xviii, xxiii, xxiv, 8, 24, 37,
    44, 60, 73, 107-110, 121
    see advocacy

# W

wages: 32, 34
wait(ing): xi, xii, xv, xvi, xxi, 19, 20,
    23, 26, 28, 40, 41, 43, 44, 46, 47,
    51, 52, 54, 55, 66, 75, 76, 82, 84,
    85, 90, 95, 101, 110, 123
whistleblower: 36, 37, 90, 117
woman: 12, 68, 84, 107, 108
    women: xv, 2, 12, 29, 45, 46, 58-
        60, 63, 98, 102, 123, 125, 128